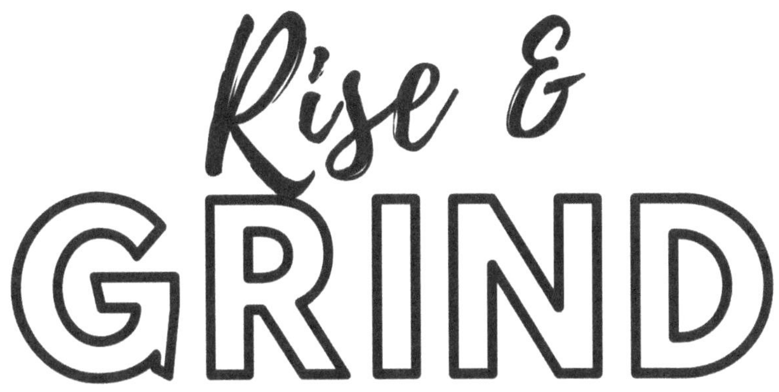

WEEKLY WORKOUT & MEAL JOURNAL

BELONGS TO:

____

____

____

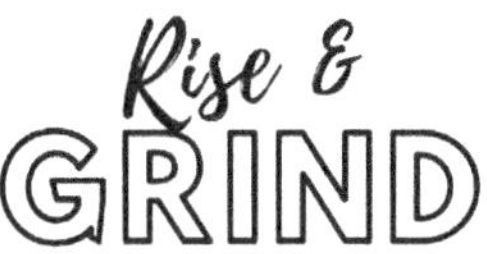

My Goals for the Year:

Goal 1:
What I'm doing about it:

Goal 2:
What I'm doing about it:

Goal 3:
What I'm doing about it:

WEEKLY MEAL PLANNER

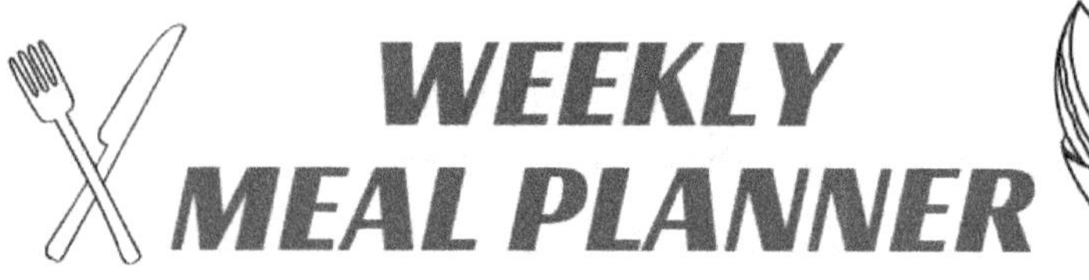

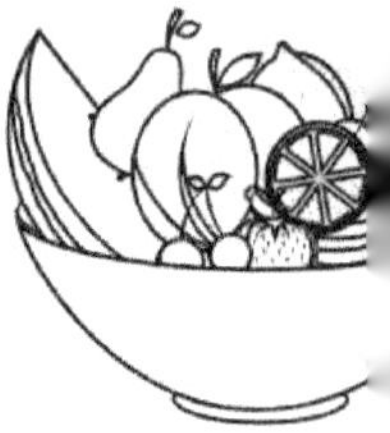

	BREAKFAST	LUNCH	SNACKS	DINNER
MONDAY				
TUESDAY				
WEDNESDAY				
THURSDSAY				
FRIDAY				
SATURDAY				
SUNDAY				

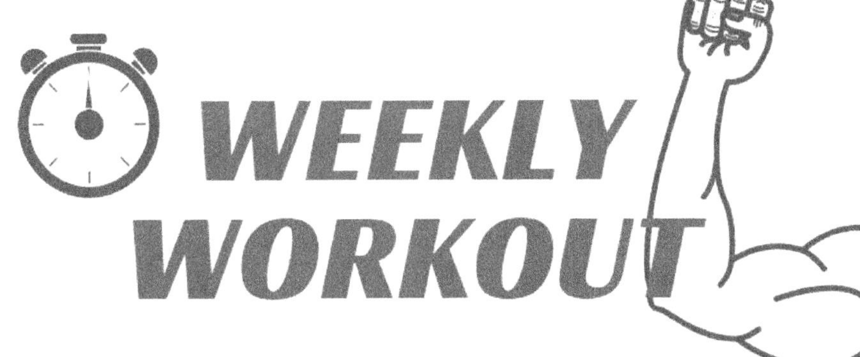

WEEKLY WORKOUT

	ACTIVITY	TIME	SETS	REPS
DAY 1				
DAY 2				
DAY 3				
DAY 4				
DAY 5				

GETTING STRONGER EVERY DAY

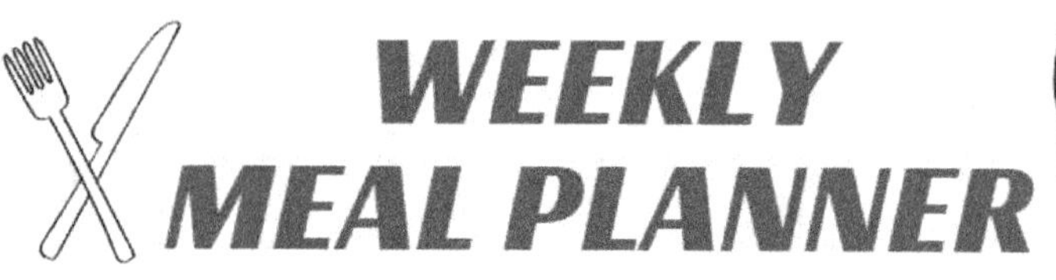

	BREAKFAST	LUNCH	SNACKS	DINNER
MONDAY				
TUESDAY				
WEDNESDAY				
THURSDSAY				
FRIDAY				
SATURDAY				
SUNDAY				

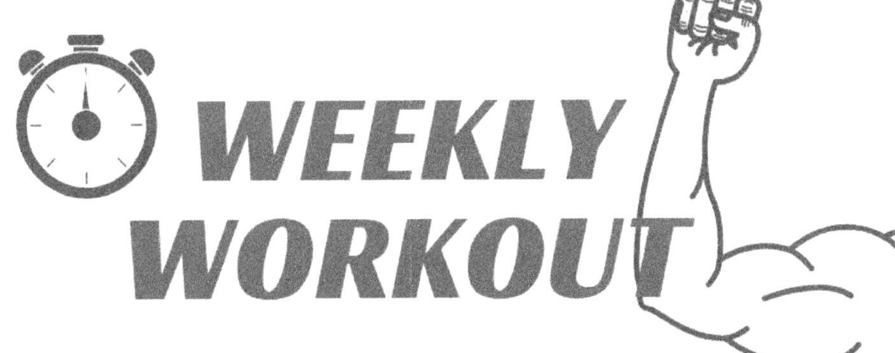

	ACTIVITY	TIME	SETS	REPS
DAY 1				
DAY 2				
DAY 3				
DAY 4				
DAY 5				

GETTING STRONGER EVERY DAY

WEEKLY MEAL PLANNER

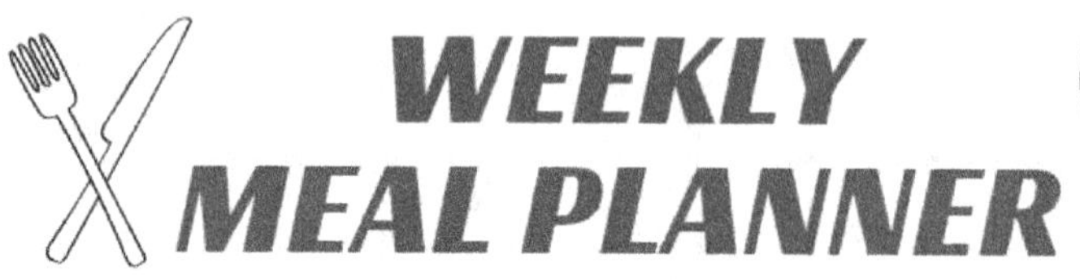
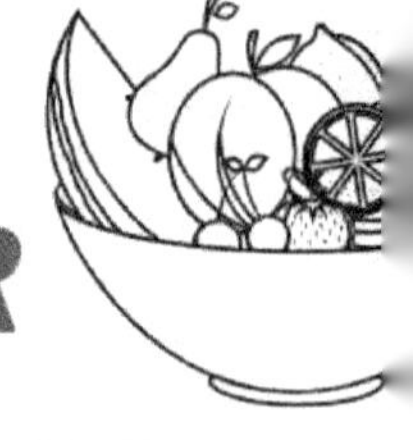

	BREAKFAST	LUNCH	SNACKS	DINNER
MONDAY				
TUESDAY				
WEDNESDAY				
THURSDSAY				
FRIDAY				
SATURDAY				
SUNDAY				

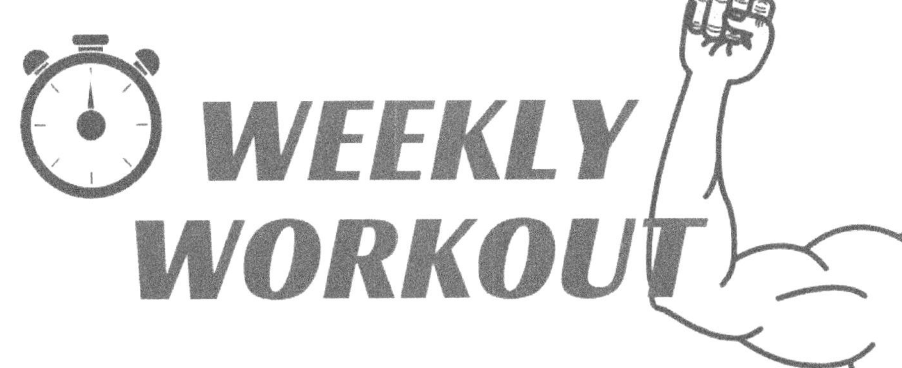

WEEKLY WORKOUT

	ACTIVITY	TIME	SETS	REPS
DAY 1				
DAY 2				
DAY 3				
DAY 4				
DAY 5				

GETTING STRONGER EVERY DAY

WEEKLY MEAL PLANNER

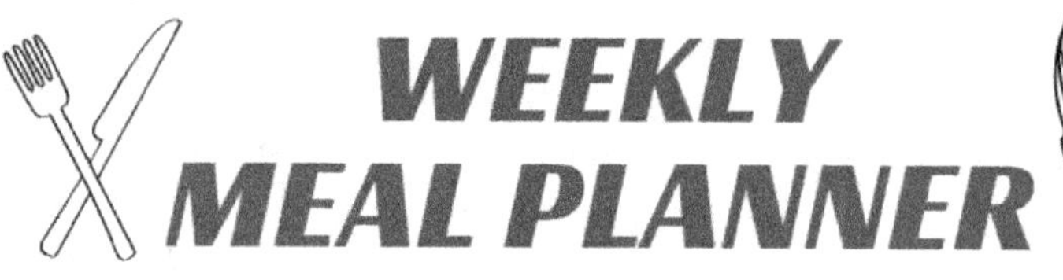
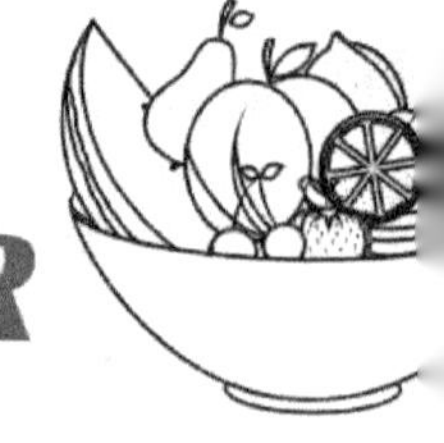

	BREAKFAST	LUNCH	SNACKS	DINNER
MONDAY				
TUESDAY				
WEDNESDAY				
THURSDSAY				
FRIDAY				
SATURDAY				
SUNDAY				

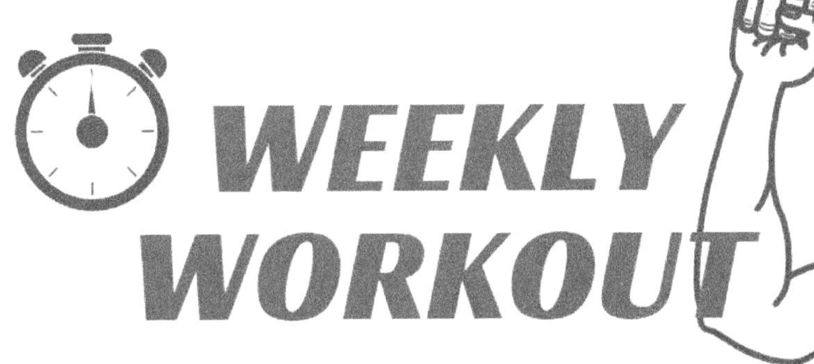

	ACTIVITY	TIME	SETS	REPS
DAY 1				
DAY 2				
DAY 3				
DAY 4				
DAY 5				

GETTING STRONGER EVERY DAY

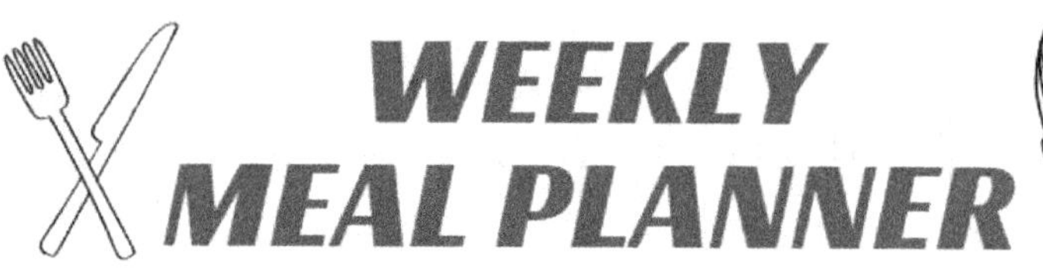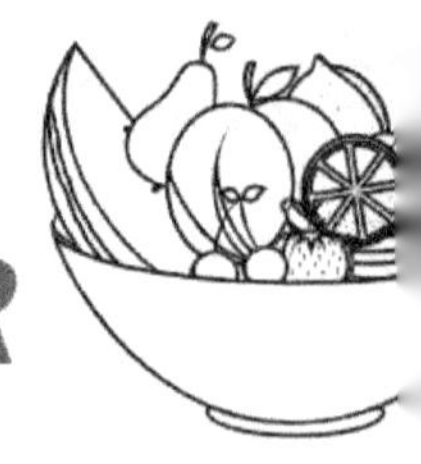

WEEKLY MEAL PLANNER

	BREAKFAST	LUNCH	SNACKS	DINNER
MONDAY				
TUESDAY				
WEDNESDAY				
THURSDSAY				
FRIDAY				
SATURDAY				
SUNDAY				

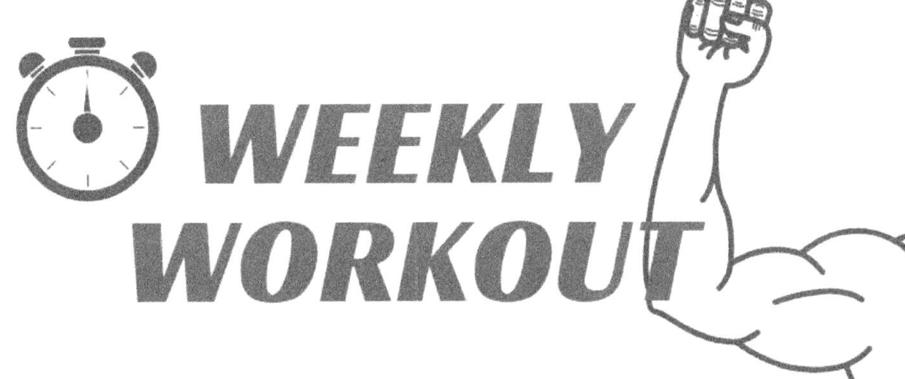

WEEKLY WORKOUT

	ACTIVITY	TIME	SETS	REPS
DAY 1				
DAY 2				
DAY 3				
DAY 4				
DAY 5				

GETTING STRONGER EVERY DAY

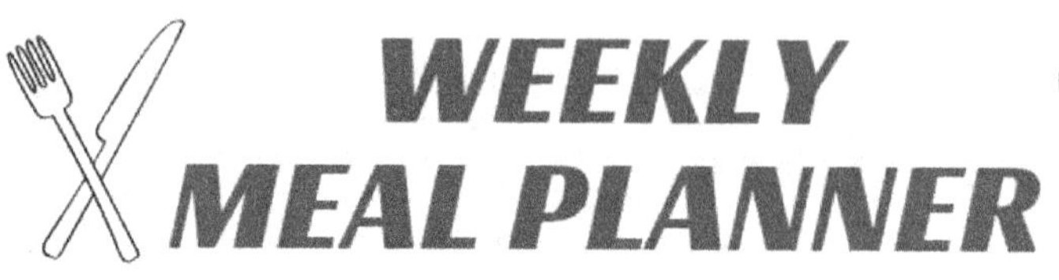

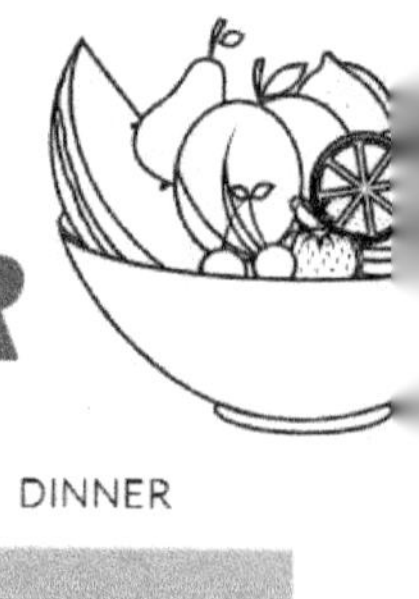

	BREAKFAST	LUNCH	SNACKS	DINNER
MONDAY				
TUESDAY				
WEDNESDAY				
THURSDSAY				
FRIDAY				
SATURDAY				
SUNDAY				

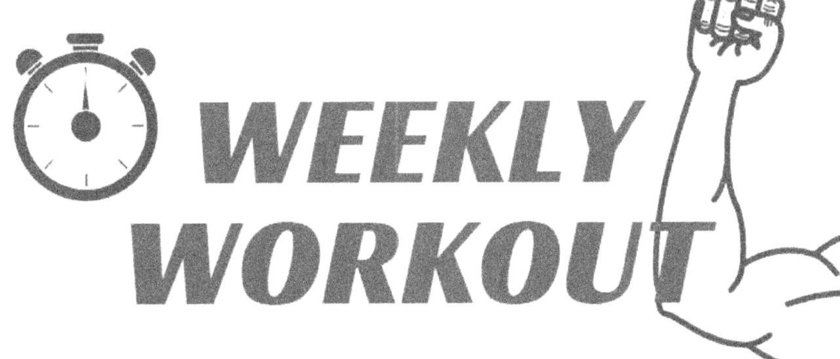

WEEKLY WORKOUT

	ACTIVITY	TIME	SETS	REPS
DAY 1				
DAY 2				
DAY 3				
DAY 4				
DAY 5				

GETTING STRONGER EVERY DAY

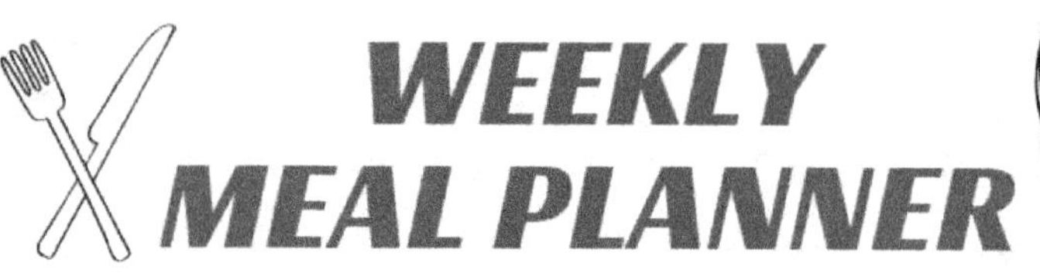 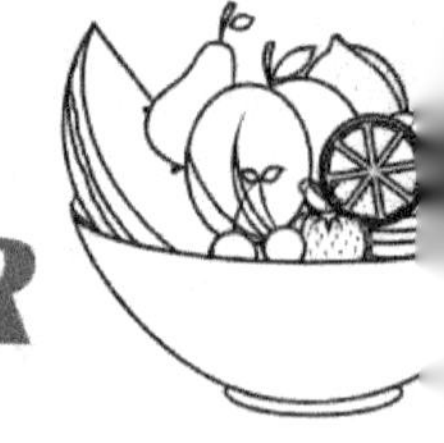

WEEKLY MEAL PLANNER

	BREAKFAST	LUNCH	SNACKS	DINNER
MONDAY				
TUESDAY				
WEDNESDAY				
THURSDSAY				
FRIDAY				
SATURDAY				
SUNDAY				

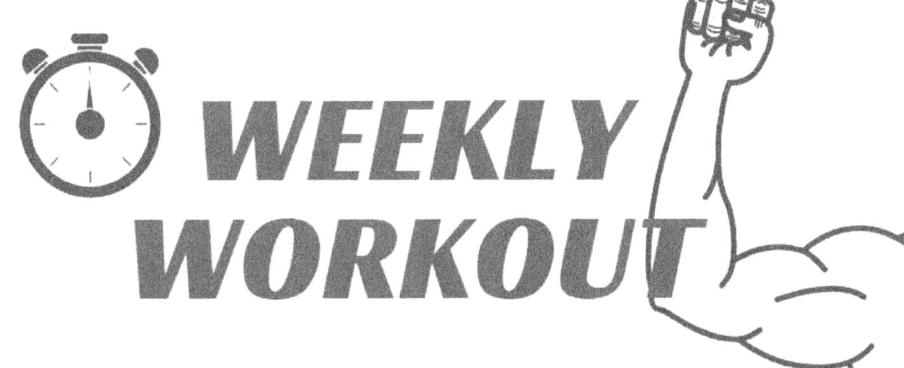

	ACTIVITY	TIME	SETS	REPS
DAY 1				
DAY 2				
DAY 3				
DAY 4				
DAY 5				

GETTING STRONGER EVERY DAY

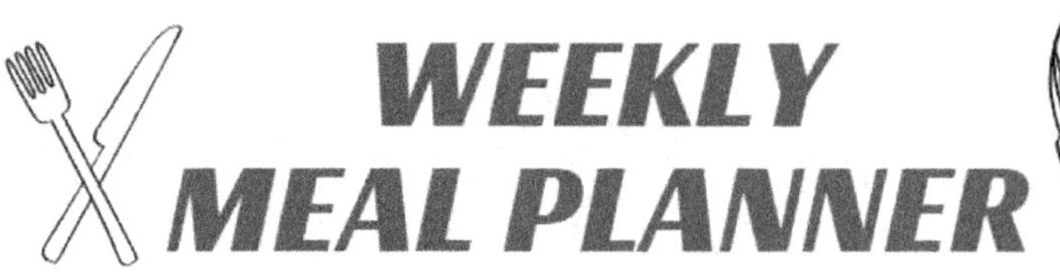 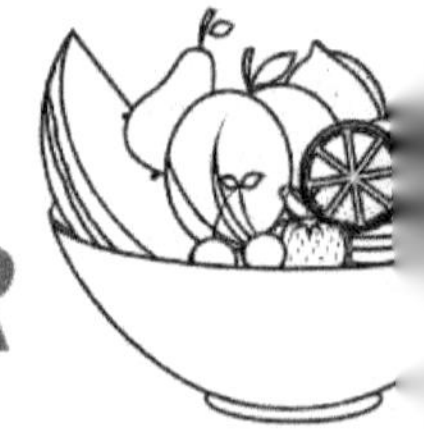

WEEKLY MEAL PLANNER

	BREAKFAST	LUNCH	SNACKS	DINNER
MONDAY				
TUESDAY				
WEDNESDAY				
THURSDSAY				
FRIDAY				
SATURDAY				
SUNDAY				

WEEKLY WORKOUT

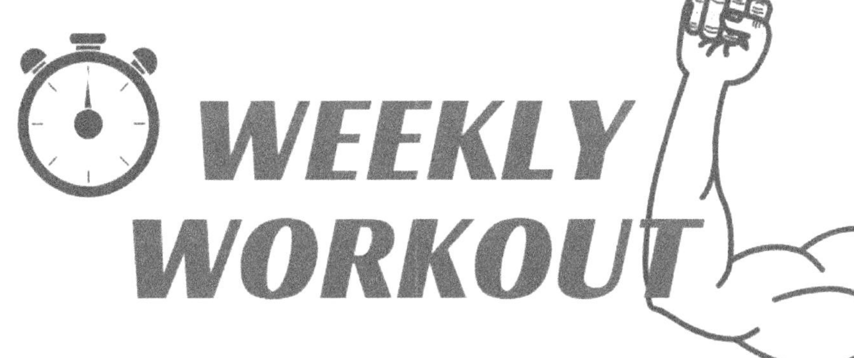

	ACTIVITY	TIME	SETS	REPS
DAY 1				
DAY 2				
DAY 3				
DAY 4				
DAY 5				

GETTING STRONGER EVERY DAY

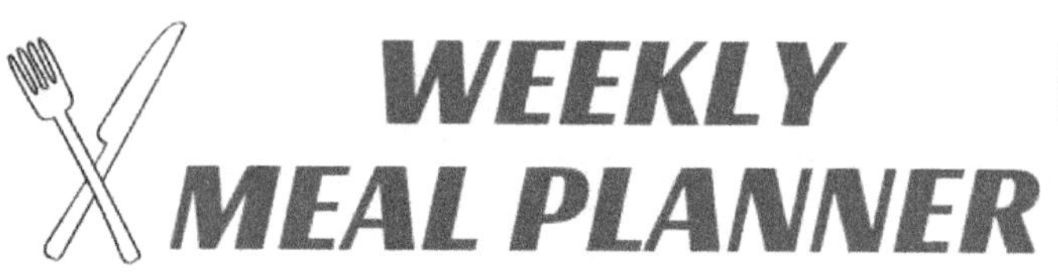

WEEKLY MEAL PLANNER

	BREAKFAST	LUNCH	SNACKS	DINNER
MONDAY				
TUESDAY				
WEDNESDAY				
THURSDSAY				
FRIDAY				
SATURDAY				
SUNDAY				

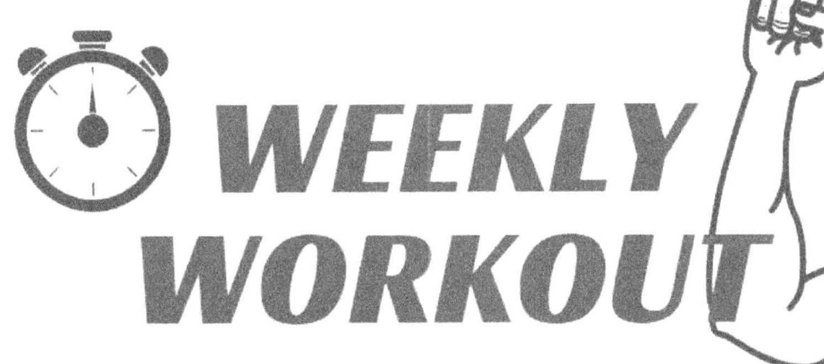

	ACTIVITY	TIME	SETS	REPS
DAY 1				
DAY 2				
DAY 3				
DAY 4				
DAY 5				

GETTING STRONGER EVERY DAY

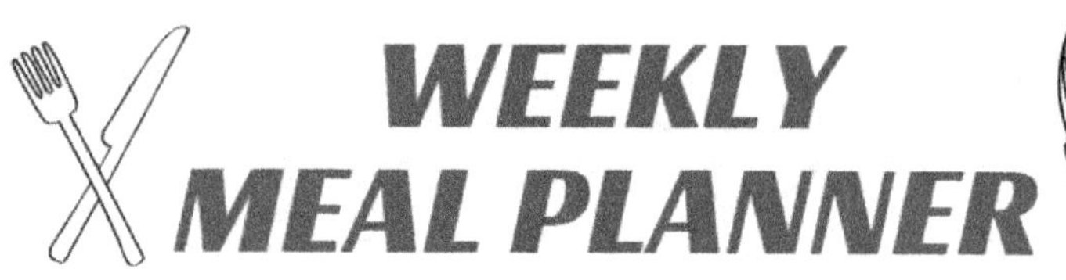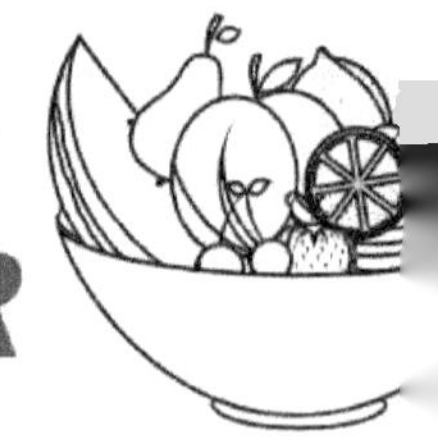

WEEKLY MEAL PLANNER

	BREAKFAST	LUNCH	SNACKS	DINNER
MONDAY				
TUESDAY				
WEDNESDAY				
THURSDSAY				
FRIDAY				
SATURDAY				
SUNDAY				

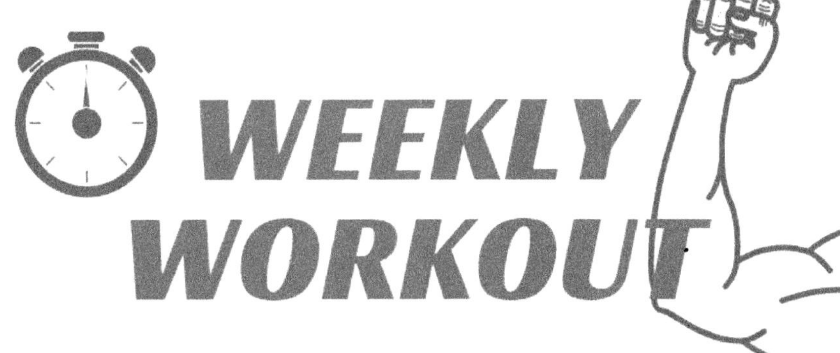

WEEKLY WORKOUT

	ACTIVITY	TIME	SETS	REPS
DAY 1				
DAY 2				
DAY 3				
DAY 4				
DAY 5				

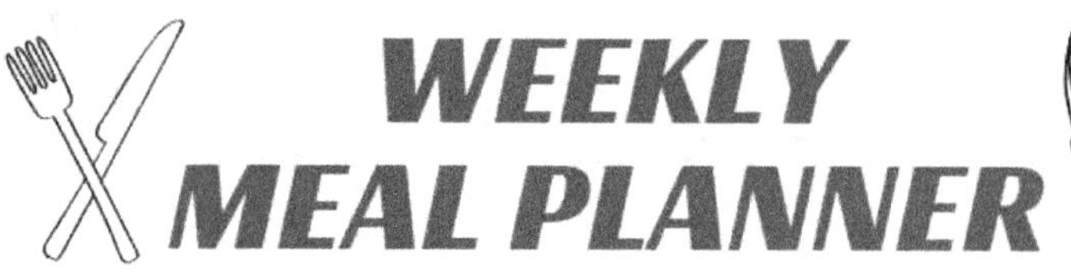

WEEKLY MEAL PLANNER

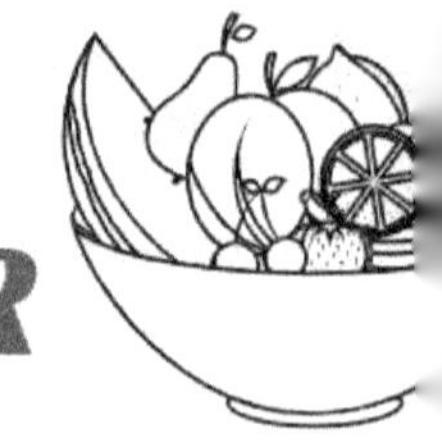

	BREAKFAST	LUNCH	SNACKS	DINNER
MONDAY				
TUESDAY				
WEDNESDAY				
THURSDSAY				
FRIDAY				
SATURDAY				
SUNDAY				

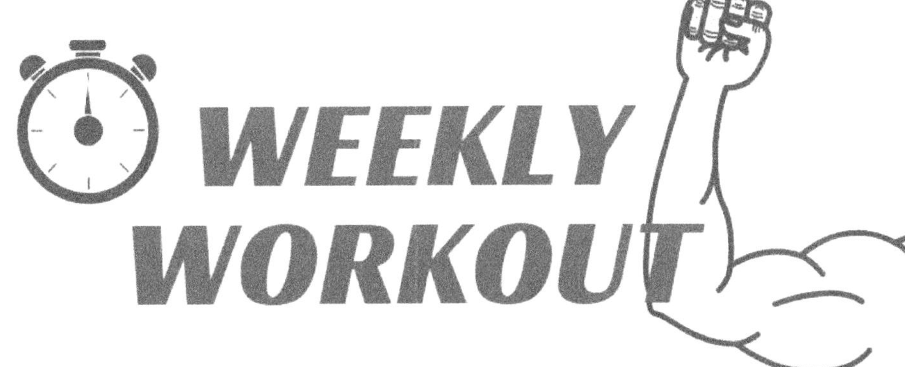

	ACTIVITY	TIME	SETS	REPS
DAY 1				
DAY 2				
DAY 3				
DAY 4				
DAY 5				

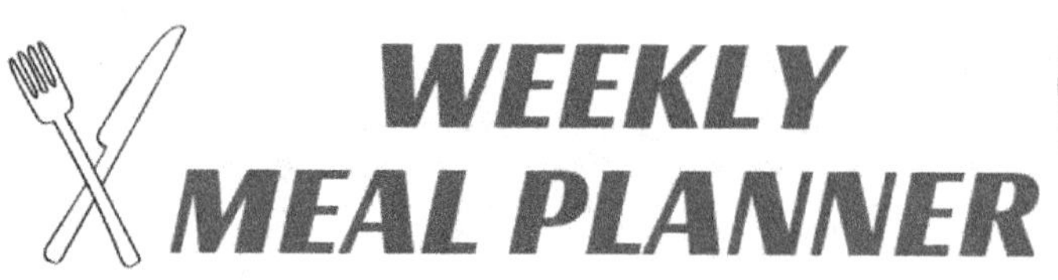

WEEKLY MEAL PLANNER

	BREAKFAST	LUNCH	SNACKS	DINNER
MONDAY				
TUESDAY				
WEDNESDAY				
THURSDSAY				
FRIDAY				
SATURDAY				
SUNDAY				

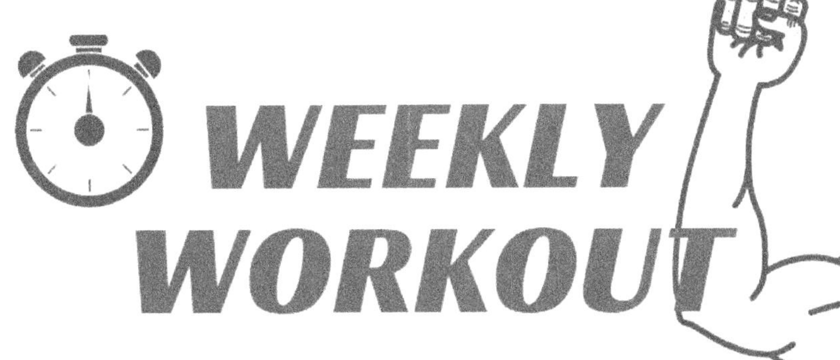

	ACTIVITY	TIME	SETS	REPS
DAY 1				
DAY 2				
DAY 3				
DAY 4				
DAY 5				

GETTING STRONGER EVERY DAY

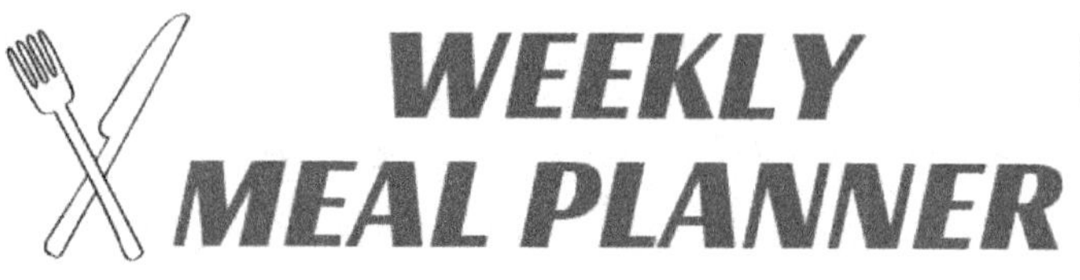
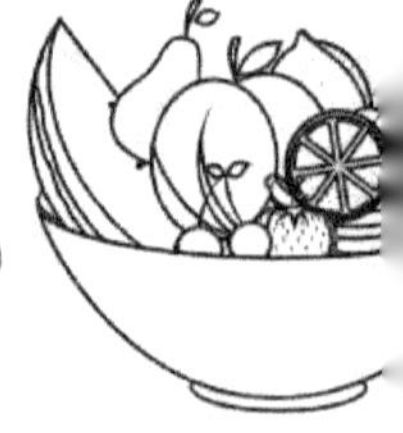

WEEKLY MEAL PLANNER

	BREAKFAST	LUNCH	SNACKS	DINNER
MONDAY				
TUESDAY				
WEDNESDAY				
THURSDSAY				
FRIDAY				
SATURDAY				
SUNDAY				

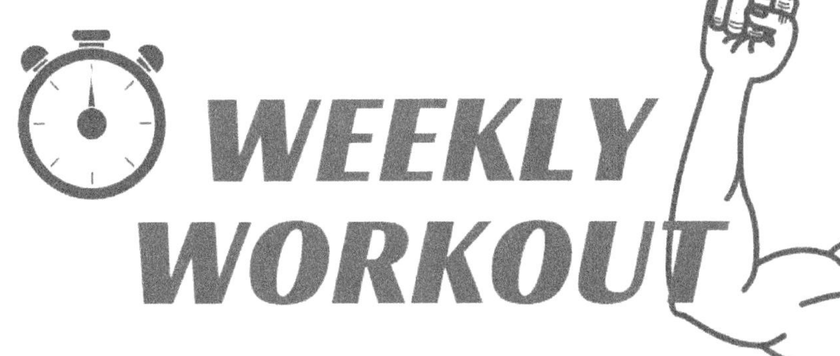

	ACTIVITY	TIME	SETS	REPS
DAY 1				
DAY 2				
DAY 3				
DAY 4				
DAY 5				

GETTING STRONGER EVERY DAY

WEEKLY MEAL PLANNER

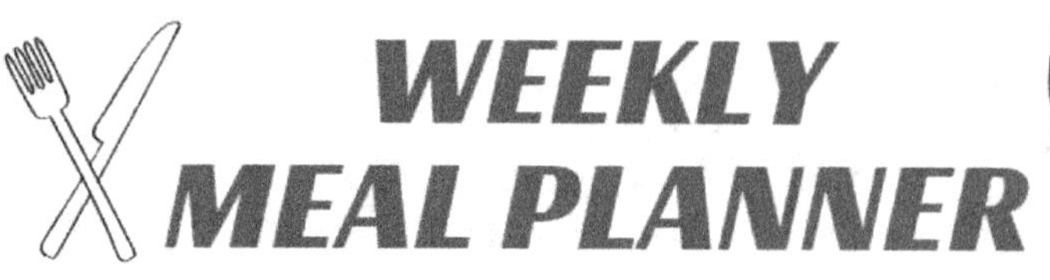

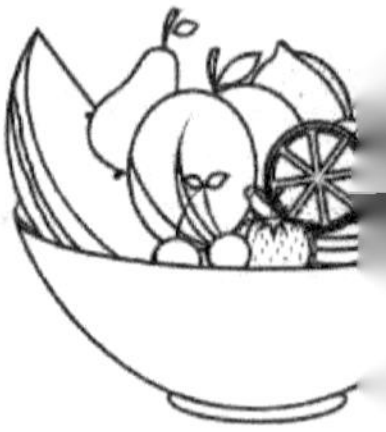

	BREAKFAST	LUNCH	SNACKS	DINNER
MONDAY				
TUESDAY				
WEDNESDAY				
THURSDSAY				
FRIDAY				
SATURDAY				
SUNDAY				

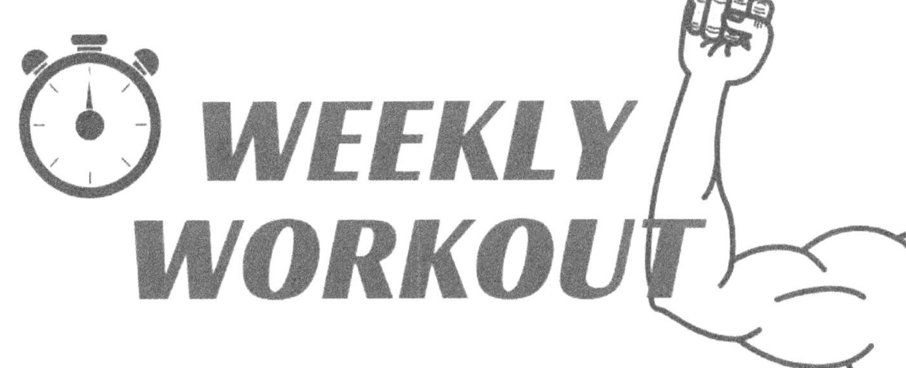

	ACTIVITY	TIME	SETS	REPS
DAY 1				
DAY 2				
DAY 3				
DAY 4				
DAY 5				

GETTING STRONGER EVERY DAY

WEEKLY MEAL PLANNER

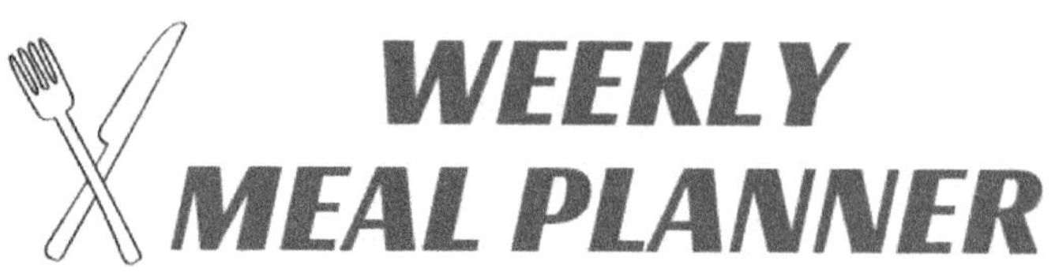

	BREAKFAST	LUNCH	SNACKS	DINNER
MONDAY				
TUESDAY				
WEDNESDAY				
THURSDSAY				
FRIDAY				
SATURDAY				
SUNDAY				

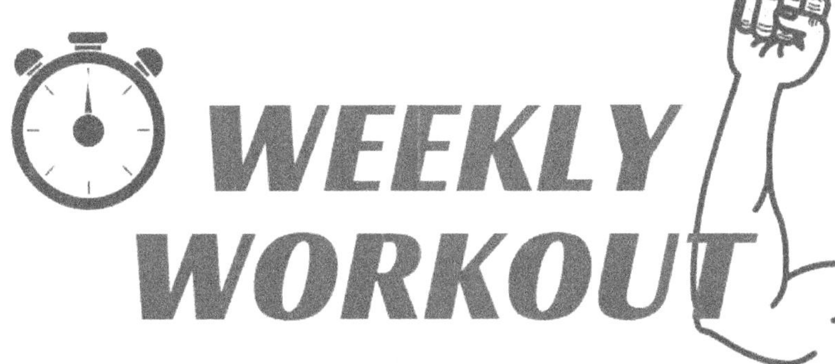

	ACTIVITY	TIME	SETS	REPS
DAY 1				
DAY 2				
DAY 3				
DAY 4				
DAY 5				

GETTING STRONGER EVERY DAY

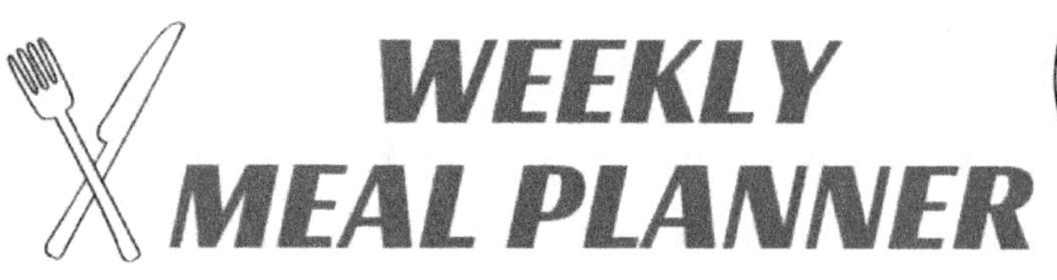

WEEKLY MEAL PLANNER

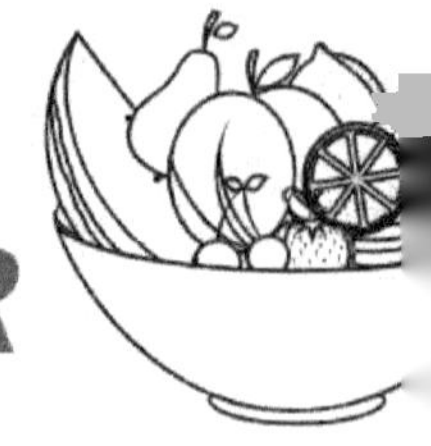

	BREAKFAST	LUNCH	SNACKS	DINNER
MONDAY				
TUESDAY				
WEDNESDAY				
THURSDSAY				
FRIDAY				
SATURDAY				
SUNDAY				

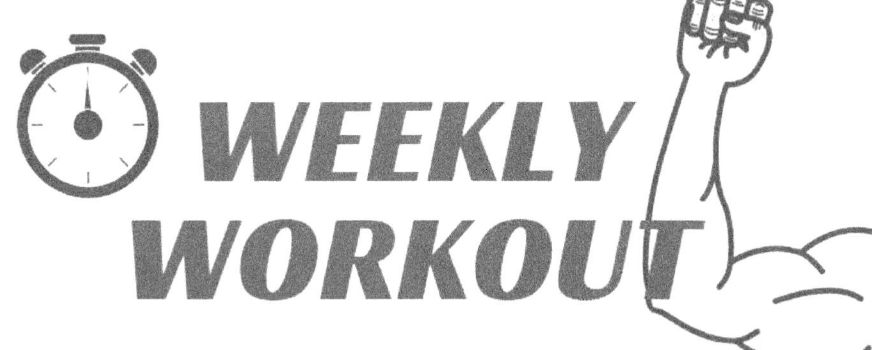

	ACTIVITY	TIME	SETS	REPS
DAY 1				
DAY 2				
DAY 3				
DAY 4				
DAY 5				

GETTING STRONGER EVERY DAY

WEEKLY MEAL PLANNER

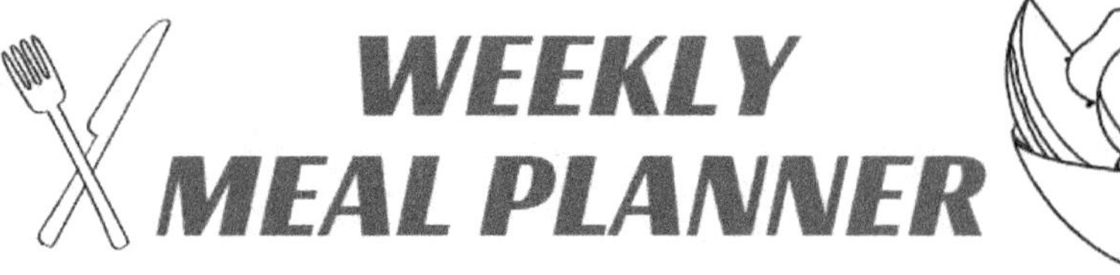

	BREAKFAST	LUNCH	SNACKS	DINNER
MONDAY				
TUESDAY				
WEDNESDAY				
THURSDSAY				
FRIDAY				
SATURDAY				
SUNDAY				

WEEKLY WORKOUT

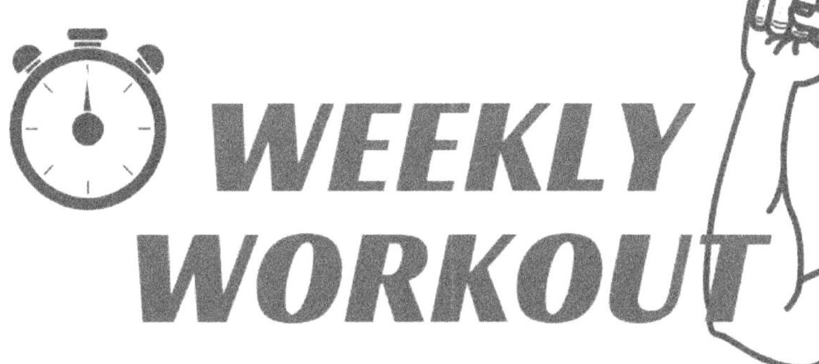

	ACTIVITY	TIME	SETS	REPS
DAY 1				
DAY 2				
DAY 3				
DAY 4				
DAY 5				

GETTING STRONGER EVERY DAY

WEEKLY MEAL PLANNER

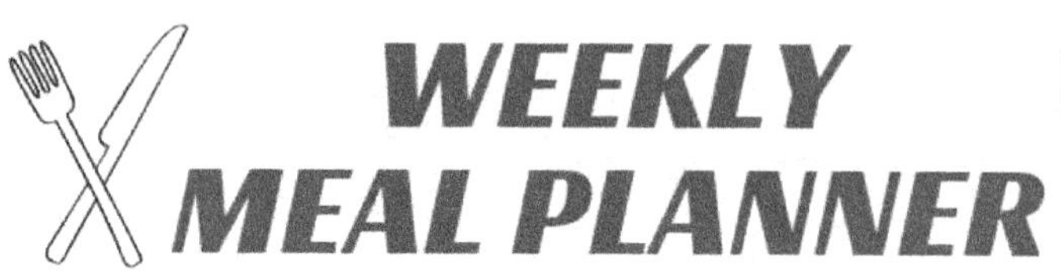

	BREAKFAST	LUNCH	SNACKS	DINNER
MONDAY				
TUESDAY				
WEDNESDAY				
THURSDSAY				
FRIDAY				
SATURDAY				
SUNDAY				

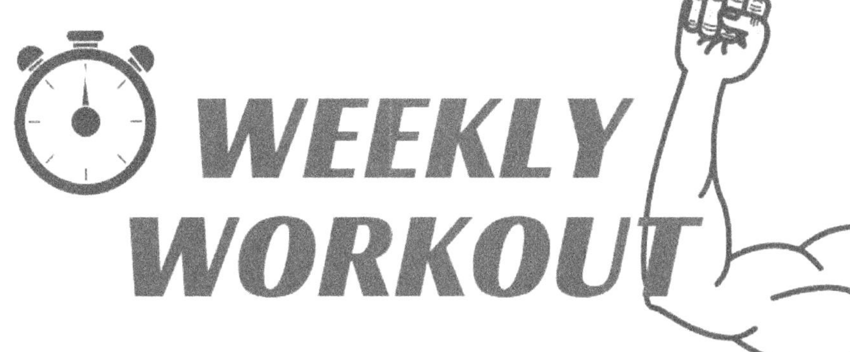

	ACTIVITY	TIME	SETS	REPS
DAY 1				
DAY 2				
DAY 3				
DAY 4				
DAY 5				

GETTING STRONGER EVERY DAY

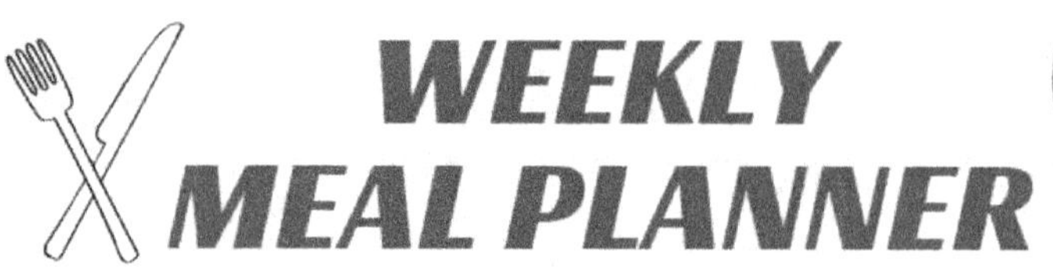

WEEKLY MEAL PLANNER

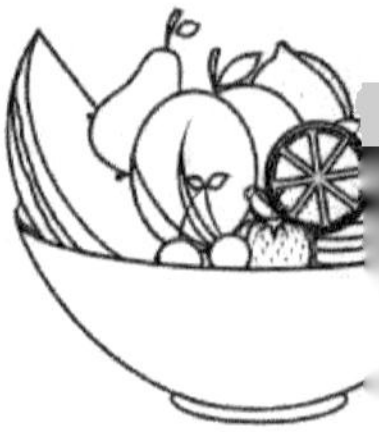

	BREAKFAST	LUNCH	SNACKS	DINNER
MONDAY				
TUESDAY				
WEDNESDAY				
THURSDSAY				
FRIDAY				
SATURDAY				
SUNDAY				

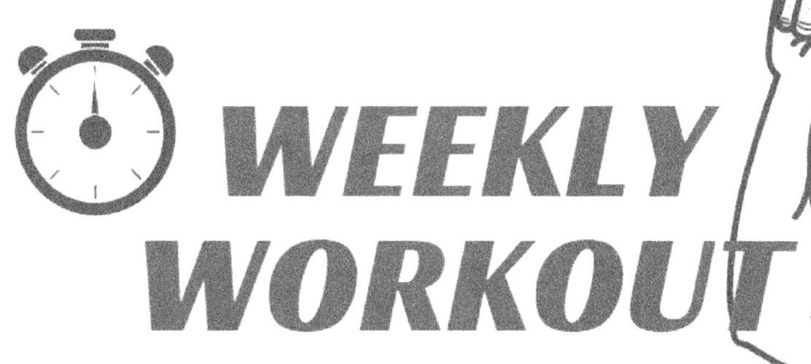

WEEKLY WORKOUT

	ACTIVITY	TIME	SETS	REPS
DAY 1				
DAY 2				
DAY 3				
DAY 4				
DAY 5				

GETTING STRONGER EVERY DAY

WEEKLY MEAL PLANNER

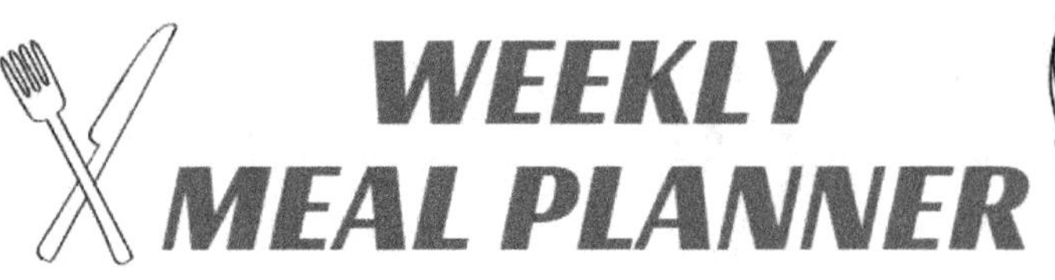

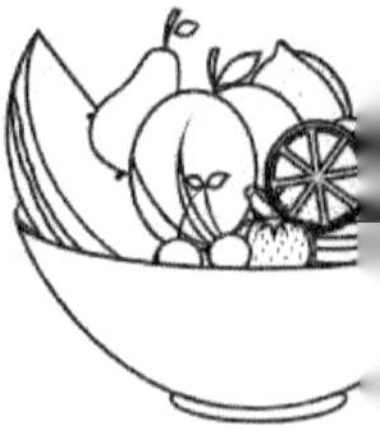

	BREAKFAST	LUNCH	SNACKS	DINNER
MONDAY				
TUESDAY				
WEDNESDAY				
THURSDSAY				
FRIDAY				
SATURDAY				
SUNDAY				

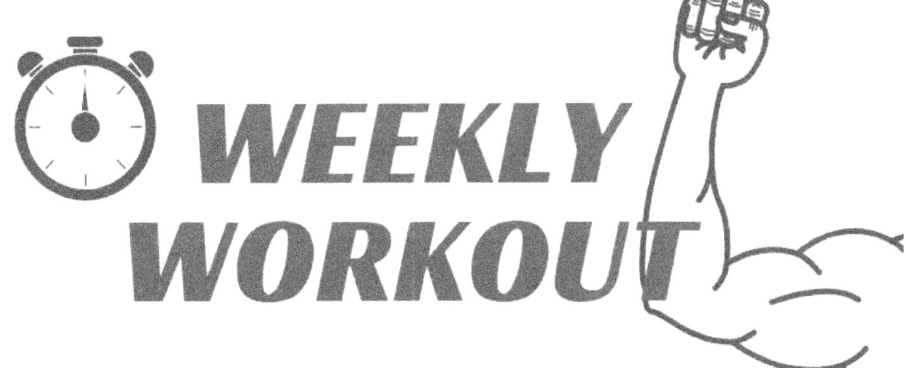

	ACTIVITY	TIME	SETS	REPS
DAY 1				
DAY 2				
DAY 3				
DAY 4				
DAY 5				

GETTING STRONGER EVERY DAY

WEEKLY MEAL PLANNER

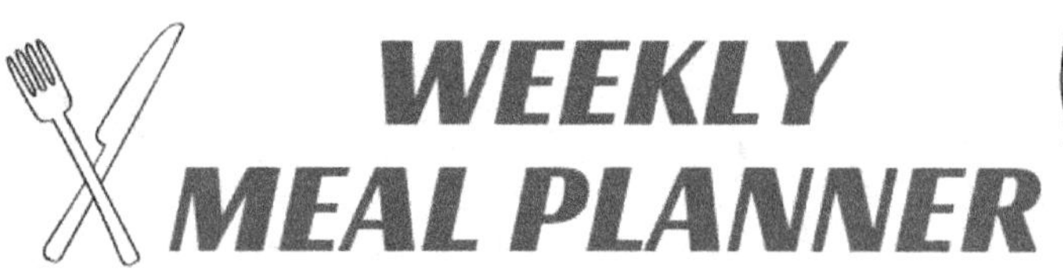

	BREAKFAST	LUNCH	SNACKS	DINNER
MONDAY				
TUESDAY				
WEDNESDAY				
THURSDSAY				
FRIDAY				
SATURDAY				
SUNDAY				

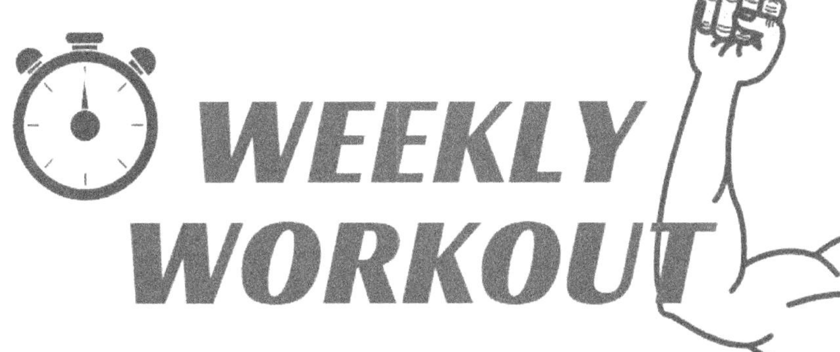

WEEKLY WORKOUT

	ACTIVITY	TIME	SETS	REPS
DAY 1				
DAY 2				
DAY 3				
DAY 4				
DAY 5				

GETTING STRONGER EVERY DAY

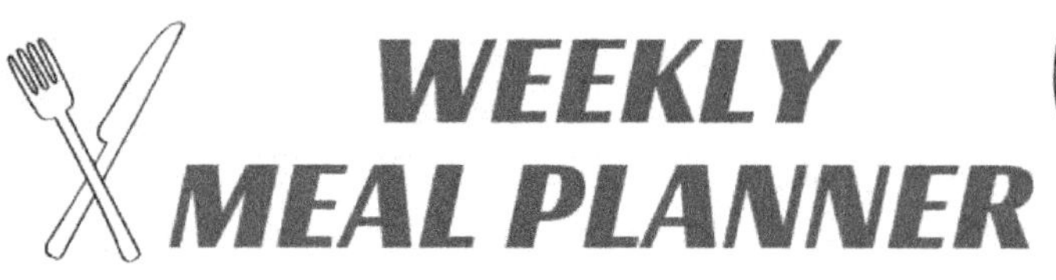 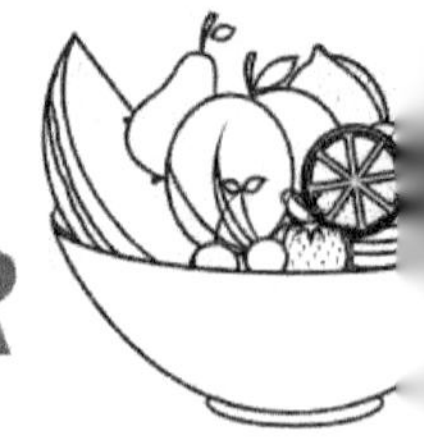

WEEKLY MEAL PLANNER

	BREAKFAST	LUNCH	SNACKS	DINNER
MONDAY				
TUESDAY				
WEDNESDAY				
THURSDSAY				
FRIDAY				
SATURDAY				
SUNDAY				

WEEKLY WORKOUT

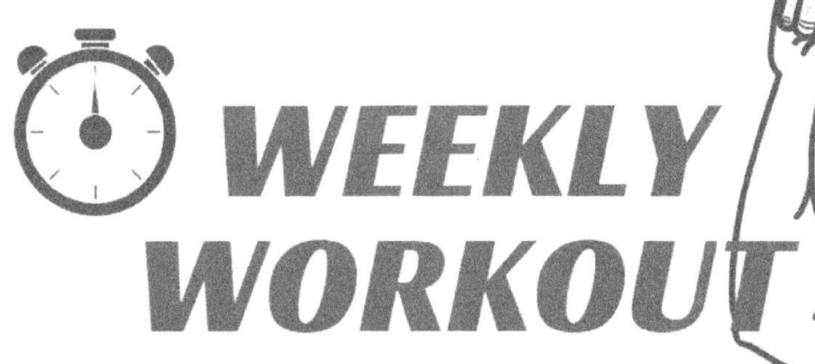

	ACTIVITY	TIME	SETS	REPS
DAY 1				
DAY 2				
DAY 3				
DAY 4				
DAY 5				

GETTING STRONGER EVERY DAY

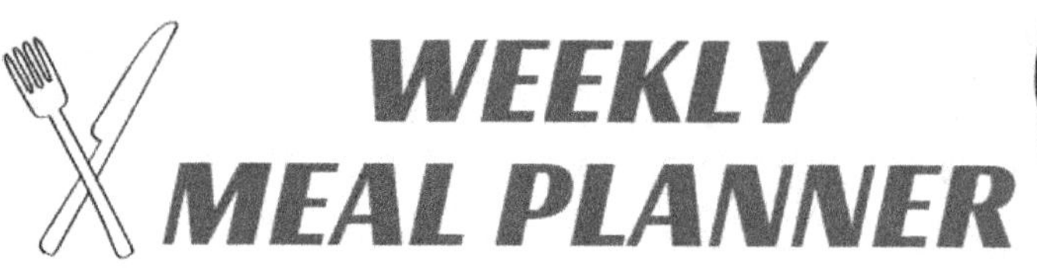
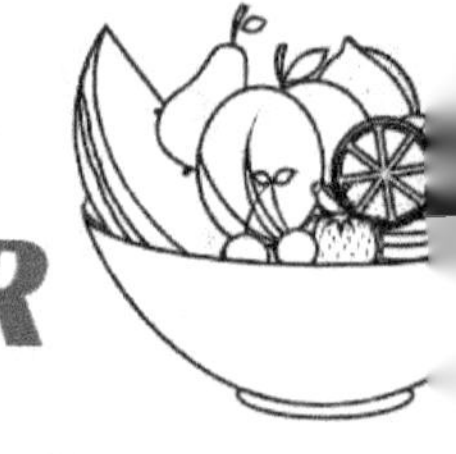

WEEKLY MEAL PLANNER

	BREAKFAST	LUNCH	SNACKS	DINNER
MONDAY				
TUESDAY				
WEDNESDAY				
THURSDSAY				
FRIDAY				
SATURDAY				
SUNDAY				

WEEKLY WORKOUT

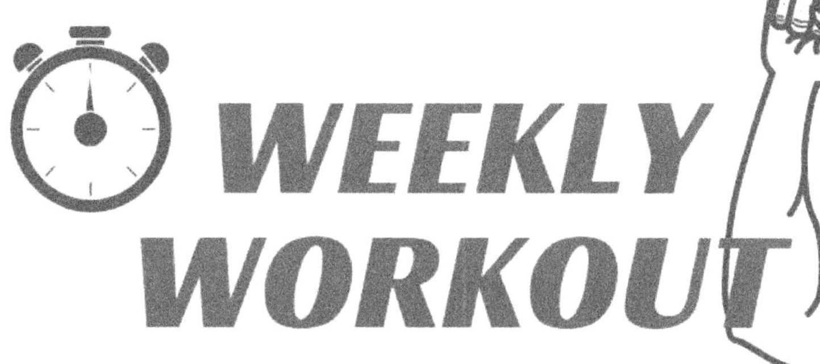

	ACTIVITY	TIME	SETS	REPS
DAY 1				
DAY 2				
DAY 3				
DAY 4				
DAY 5				

GETTING STRONGER EVERY DAY

WEEKLY MEAL PLANNER

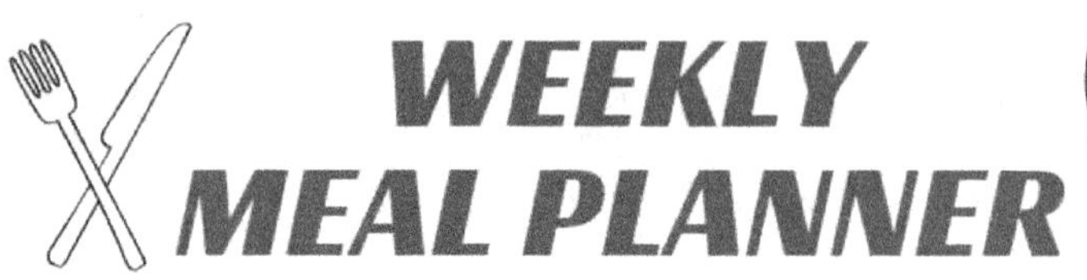

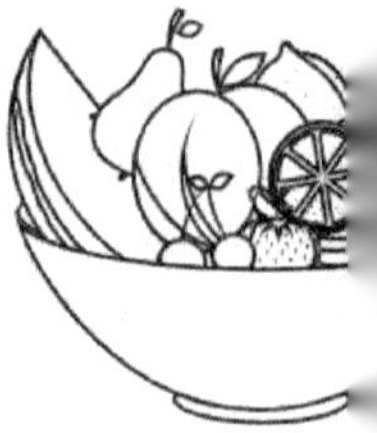

	BREAKFAST	LUNCH	SNACKS	DINNER
MONDAY				
TUESDAY				
WEDNESDAY				
THURSDSAY				
FRIDAY				
SATURDAY				
SUNDAY				

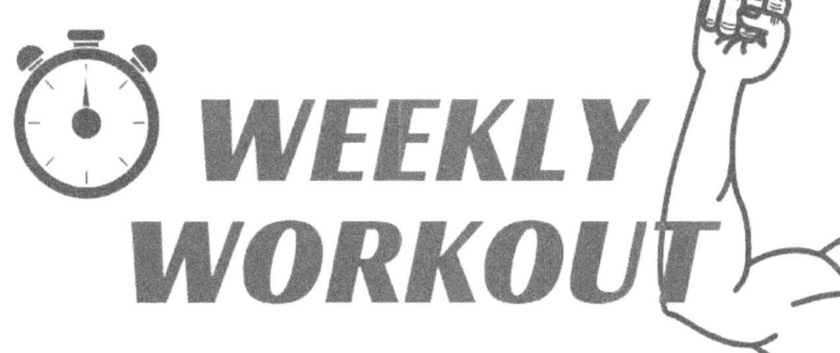

WEEKLY WORKOUT

	ACTIVITY	TIME	SETS	REPS
DAY 1				
DAY 2				
DAY 3				
DAY 4				
DAY 5				

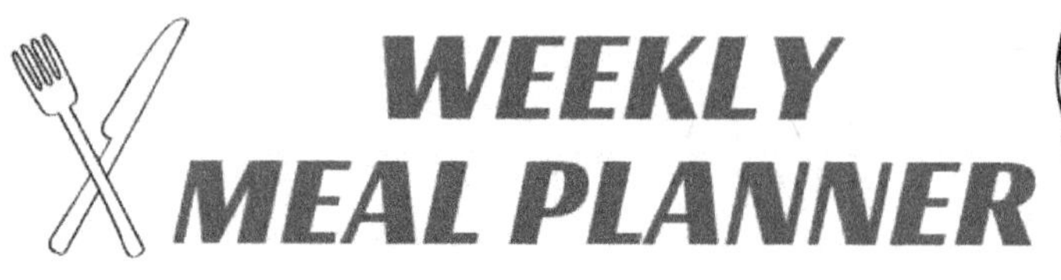

WEEKLY MEAL PLANNER

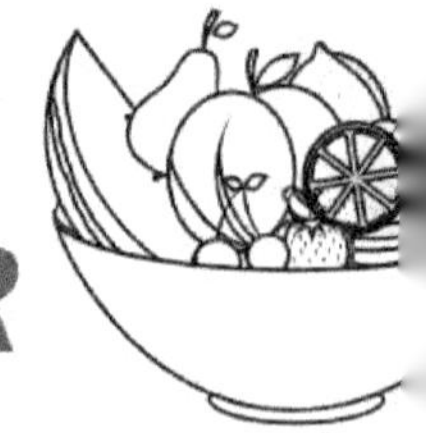

	BREAKFAST	LUNCH	SNACKS	DINNER
MONDAY				
TUESDAY				
WEDNESDAY				
THURSDSAY				
FRIDAY				
SATURDAY				
SUNDAY				

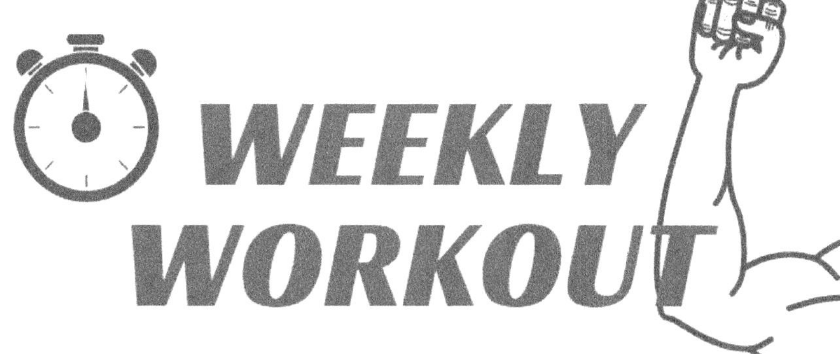

	ACTIVITY	TIME	SETS	REPS
DAY 1				
DAY 2				
DAY 3				
DAY 4				
DAY 5				

GETTING STRONGER EVERY DAY

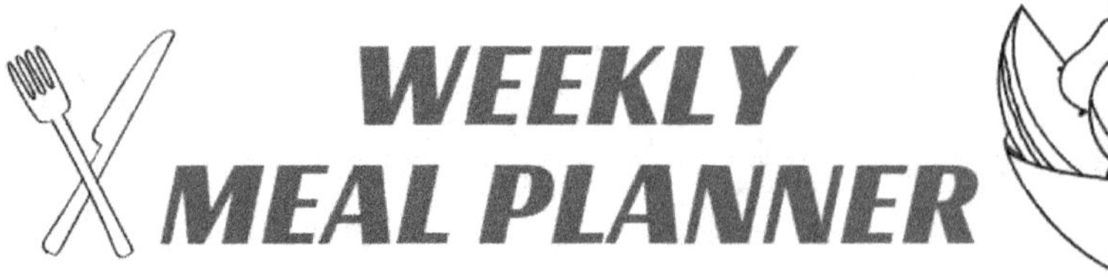

	BREAKFAST	LUNCH	SNACKS	DINNER
MONDAY				
TUESDAY				
WEDNESDAY				
THURSDSAY				
FRIDAY				
SATURDAY				
SUNDAY				

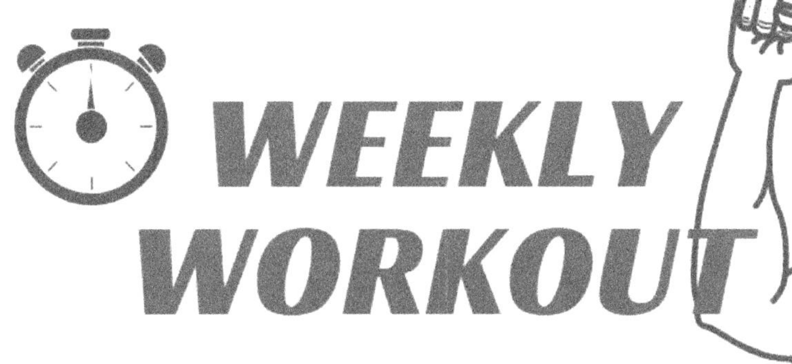

WEEKLY WORKOUT

	ACTIVITY	TIME	SETS	REPS
DAY 1				
DAY 2				
DAY 3				
DAY 4				
DAY 5				

GETTING STRONGER EVERY DAY

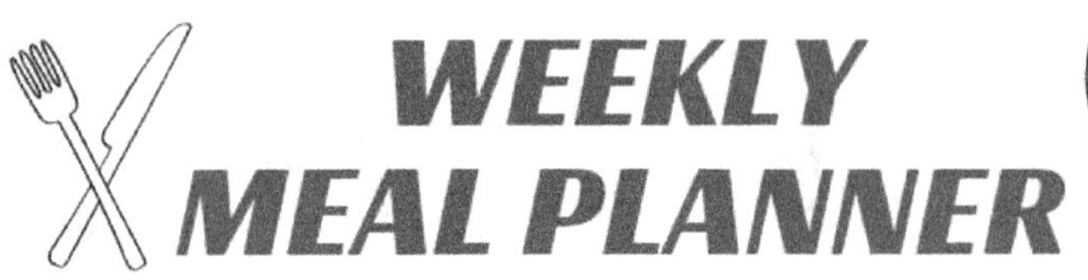

WEEKLY MEAL PLANNER

	BREAKFAST	LUNCH	SNACKS	DINNER
MONDAY				
TUESDAY				
WEDNESDAY				
THURSDSAY				
FRIDAY				
SATURDAY				
SUNDAY				

WEEKLY WORKOUT

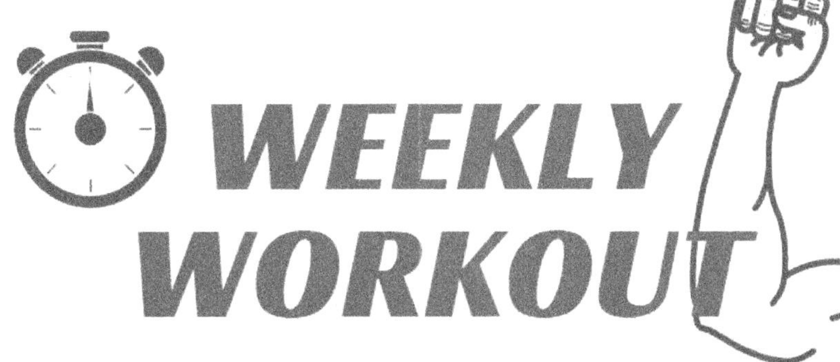

	ACTIVITY	TIME	SETS	REPS
DAY 1				
DAY 2				
DAY 3				
DAY 4				
DAY 5				

GETTING STRONGER EVERY DAY

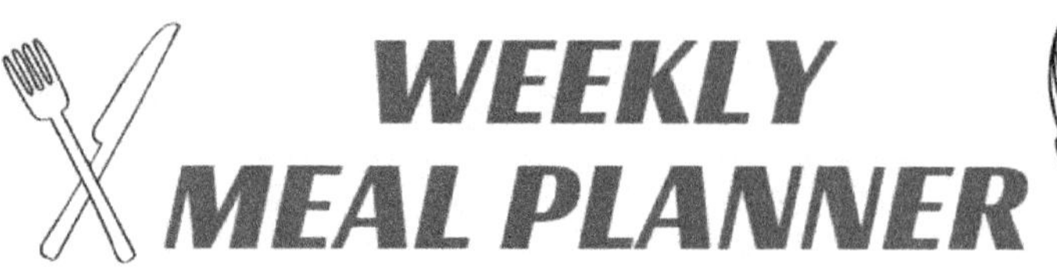
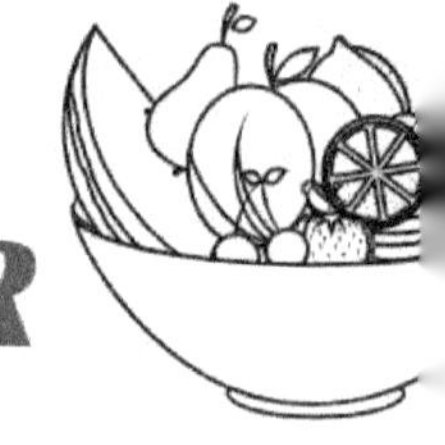

WEEKLY MEAL PLANNER

	BREAKFAST	LUNCH	SNACKS	DINNER
MONDAY				
TUESDAY				
WEDNESDAY				
THURSDSAY				
FRIDAY				
SATURDAY				
SUNDAY				

WEEKLY WORKOUT

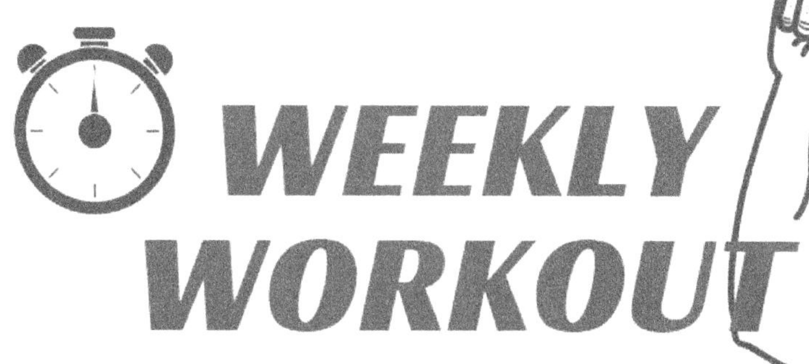

	ACTIVITY	TIME	SETS	REPS
DAY 1				
DAY 2				
DAY 3				
DAY 4				
DAY 5				

GETTING STRONGER EVERY DAY

WEEKLY MEAL PLANNER

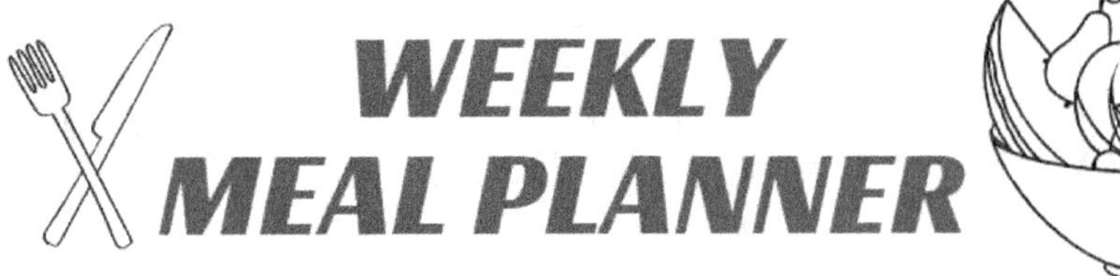

	BREAKFAST	LUNCH	SNACKS	DINNER
MONDAY				
TUESDAY				
WEDNESDAY				
THURSDSAY				
FRIDAY				
SATURDAY				
SUNDAY				

WEEKLY WORKOUT

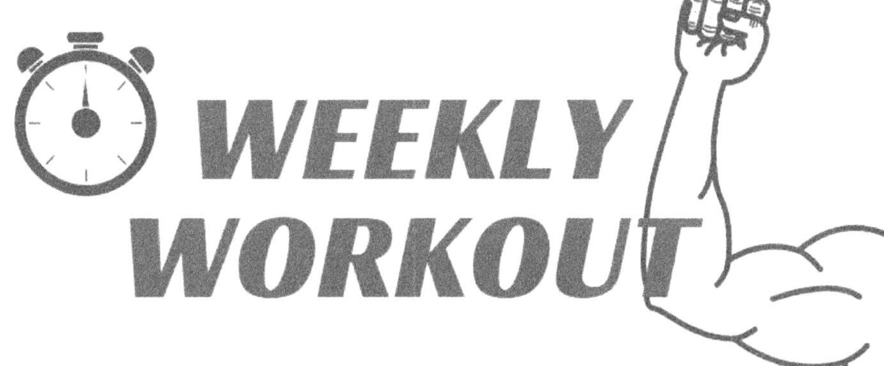

	ACTIVITY	TIME	SETS	REPS
DAY 1				
DAY 2				
DAY 3				
DAY 4				
DAY 5				

GETTING STRONGER EVERY DAY

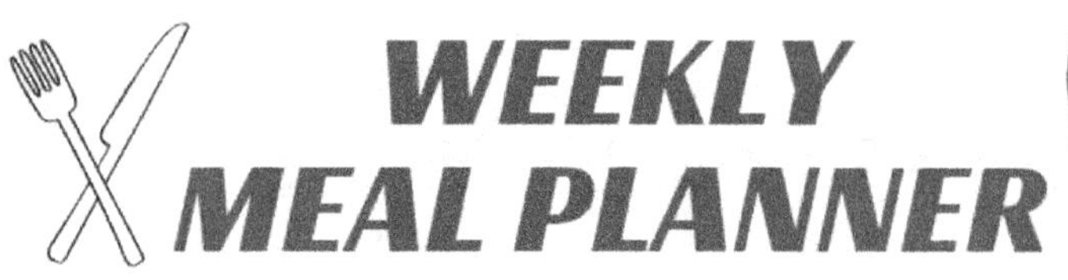

WEEKLY MEAL PLANNER

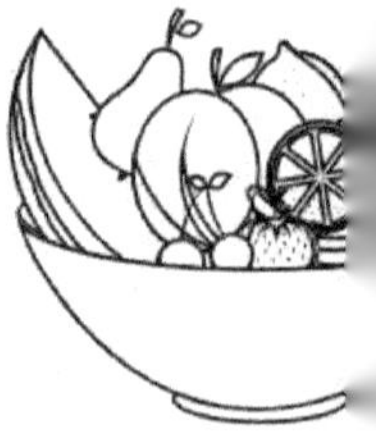

	BREAKFAST	LUNCH	SNACKS	DINNER
MONDAY				
TUESDAY				
WEDNESDAY				
THURSDSAY				
FRIDAY				
SATURDAY				
SUNDAY				

WEEKLY WORKOUT

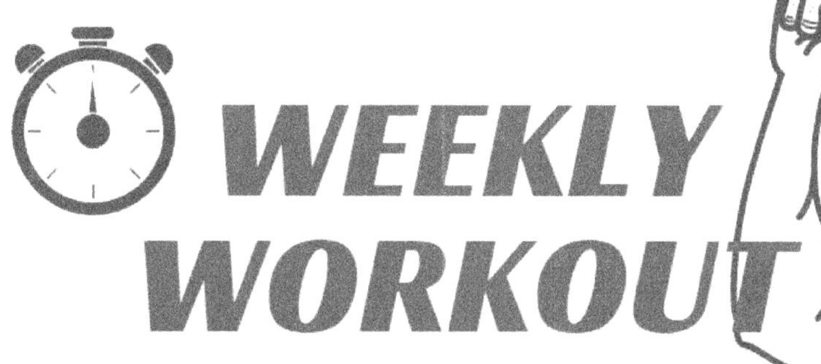

	ACTIVITY	TIME	SETS	REPS
DAY 1				
DAY 2				
DAY 3				
DAY 4				
DAY 5				

GETTING STRONGER EVERY DAY

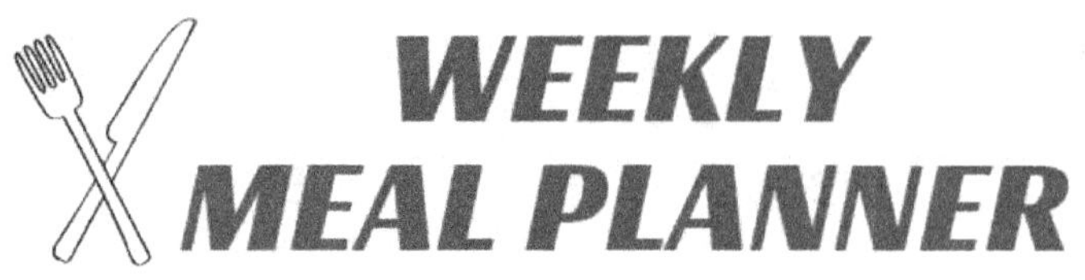

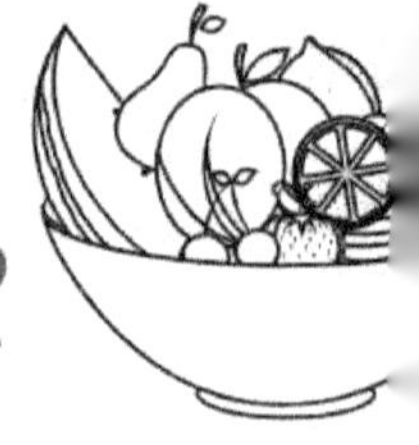

	BREAKFAST	LUNCH	SNACKS	DINNER
MONDAY				
TUESDAY				
WEDNESDAY				
THURSDSAY				
FRIDAY				
SATURDAY				
SUNDAY				

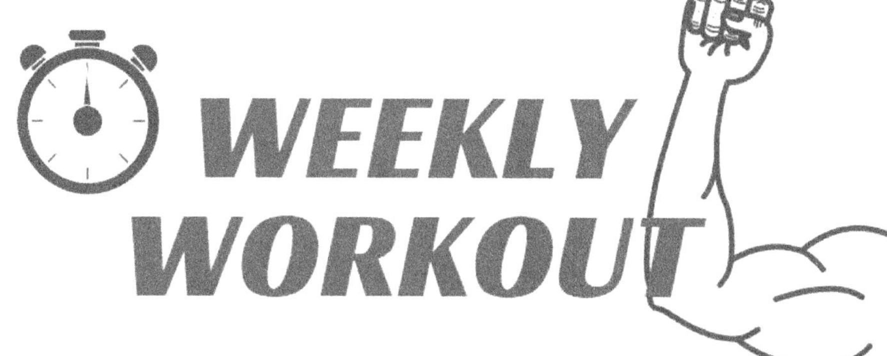

	ACTIVITY	TIME	SETS	REPS
DAY 1				
DAY 2				
DAY 3				
DAY 4				
DAY 5				

GETTING STRONGER EVERY DAY

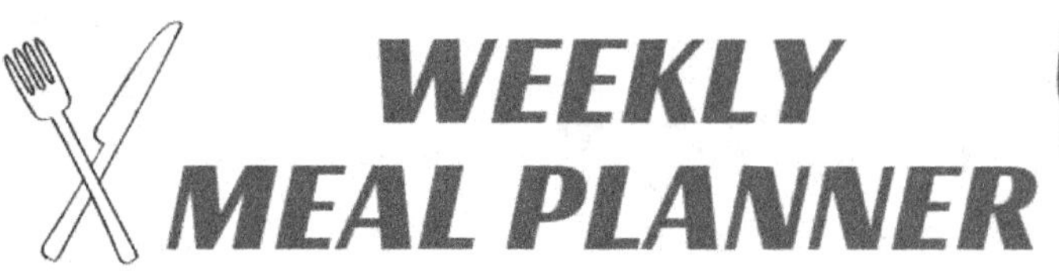
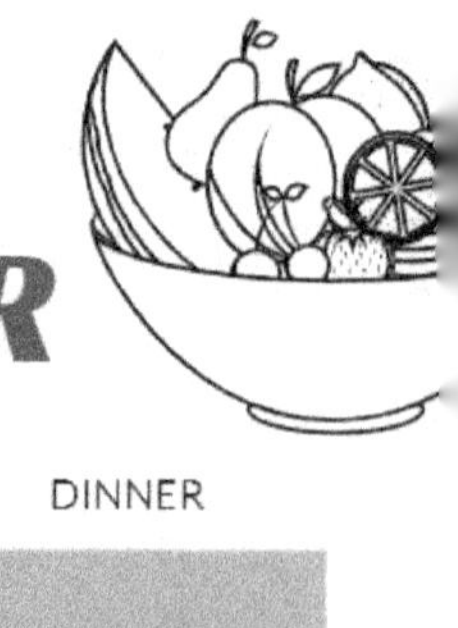

WEEKLY MEAL PLANNER

	BREAKFAST	LUNCH	SNACKS	DINNER
MONDAY				
TUESDAY				
WEDNESDAY				
THURSDSAY				
FRIDAY				
SATURDAY				
SUNDAY				

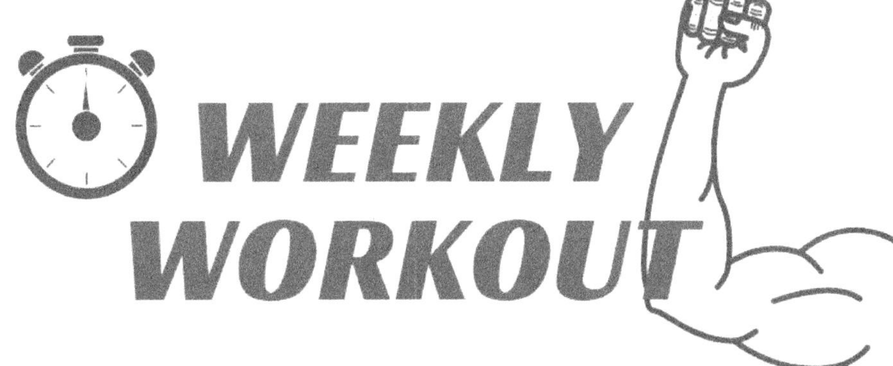

	ACTIVITY	TIME	SETS	REPS
DAY 1				
DAY 2				
DAY 3				
DAY 4				
DAY 5				

GETTING STRONGER EVERY DAY

WEEKLY MEAL PLANNER

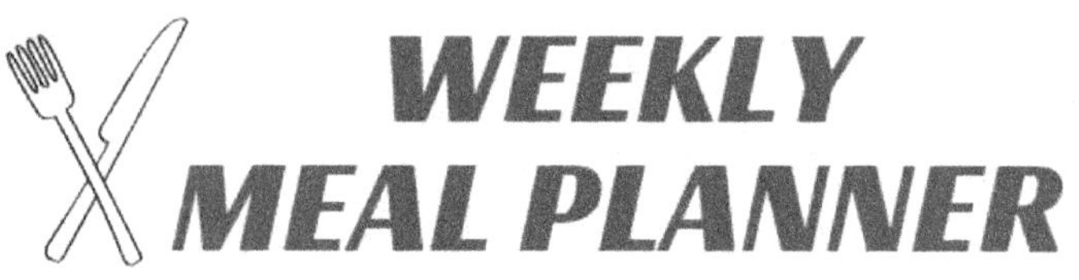

	BREAKFAST	LUNCH	SNACKS	DINNER
MONDAY				
TUESDAY				
WEDNESDAY				
THURSDSAY				
FRIDAY				
SATURDAY				
SUNDAY				

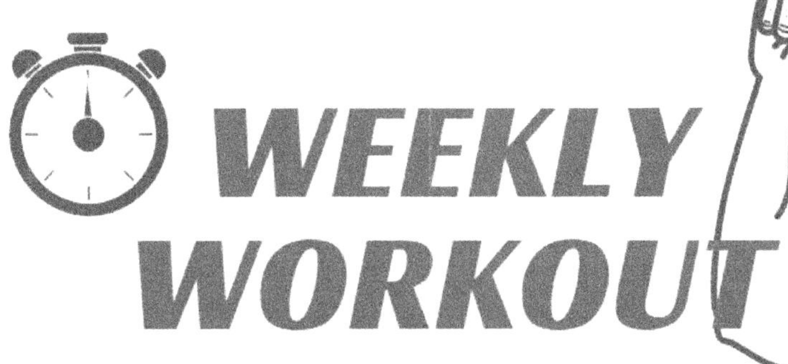

	ACTIVITY	TIME	SETS	REPS
DAY 1				
DAY 2				
DAY 3				
DAY 4				
DAY 5				

GETTING STRONGER EVERY DAY

WEEKLY MEAL PLANNER

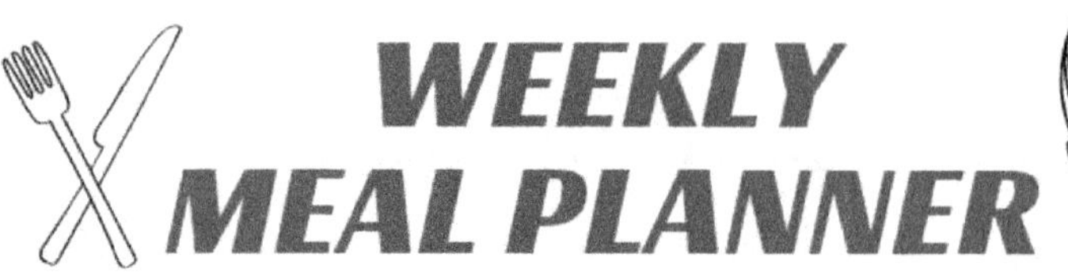

	BREAKFAST	LUNCH	SNACKS	DINNER
MONDAY				
TUESDAY				
WEDNESDAY				
THURSDSAY				
FRIDAY				
SATURDAY				
SUNDAY				

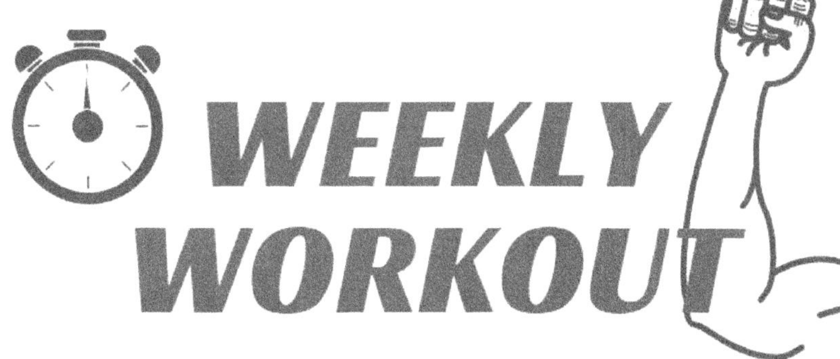

WEEKLY WORKOUT

	ACTIVITY	TIME	SETS	REPS
DAY 1				
DAY 2				
DAY 3				
DAY 4				
DAY 5				

GETTING STRONGER EVERY DAY

WEEKLY MEAL PLANNER

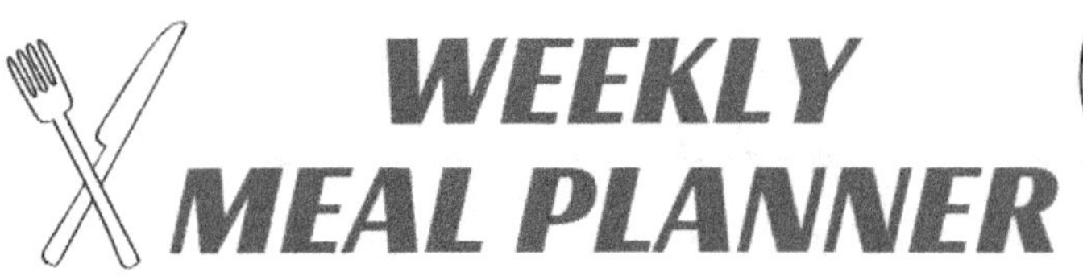

	BREAKFAST	LUNCH	SNACKS	DINNER
MONDAY				
TUESDAY				
WEDNESDAY				
THURSDSAY				
FRIDAY				
SATURDAY				
SUNDAY				

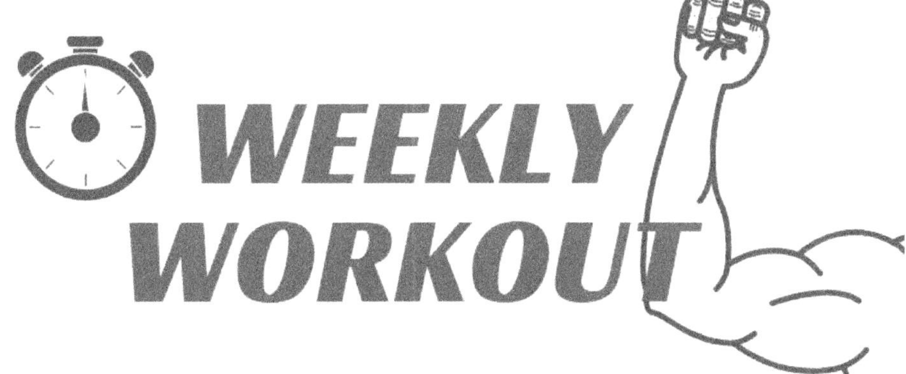

ACTIVITY	TIME	SETS	REPS
DAY 1			
DAY 2			
DAY 3			
DAY 4			
DAY 5			

GETTING STRONGER EVERY DAY

WEEKLY MEAL PLANNER

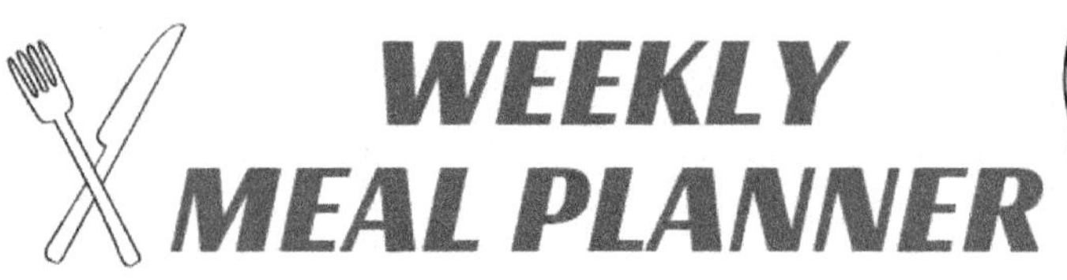

	BREAKFAST	LUNCH	SNACKS	DINNER
MONDAY				
TUESDAY				
WEDNESDAY				
THURSDSAY				
FRIDAY				
SATURDAY				
SUNDAY				

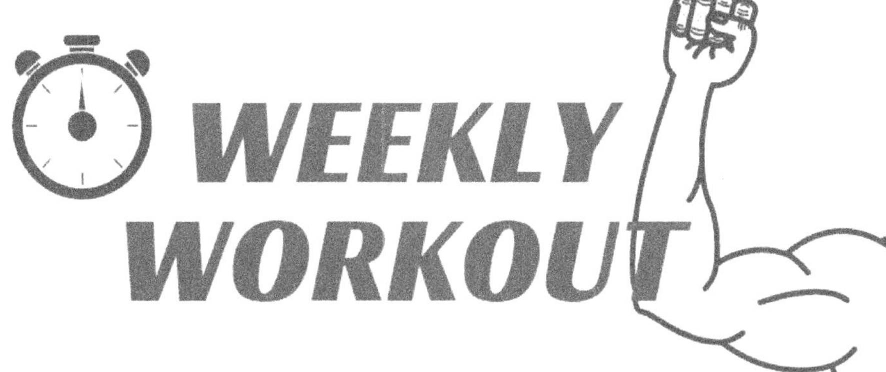

	ACTIVITY	TIME	SETS	REPS
DAY 1				
DAY 2				
DAY 3				
DAY 4				
DAY 5				

GETTING STRONGER EVERY DAY

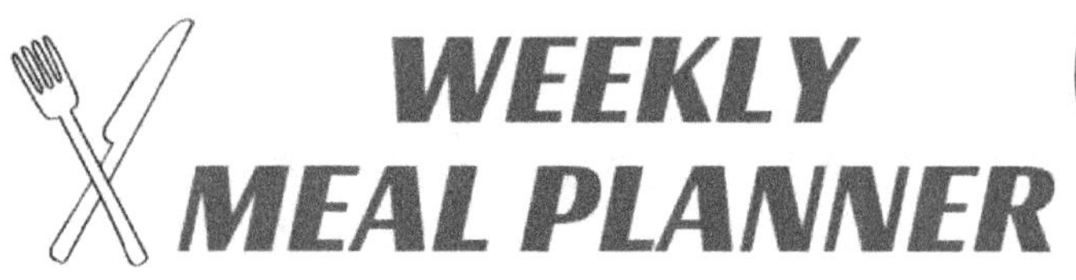

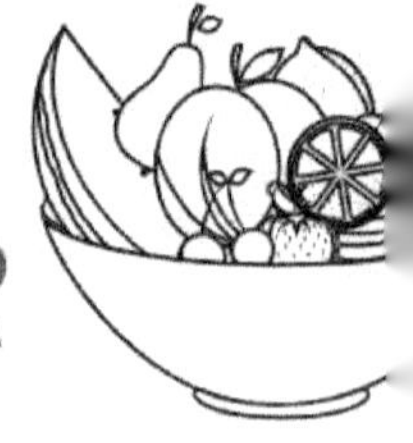

	BREAKFAST	LUNCH	SNACKS	DINNER
MONDAY				
TUESDAY				
WEDNESDAY				
THURSDSAY				
FRIDAY				
SATURDAY				
SUNDAY				

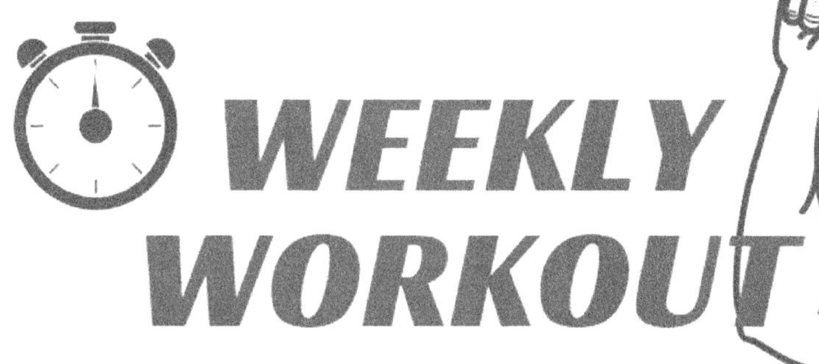

WEEKLY WORKOUT

ACTIVITY	TIME	SETS	REPS
DAY 1			
DAY 2			
DAY 3			
DAY 4			
DAY 5			

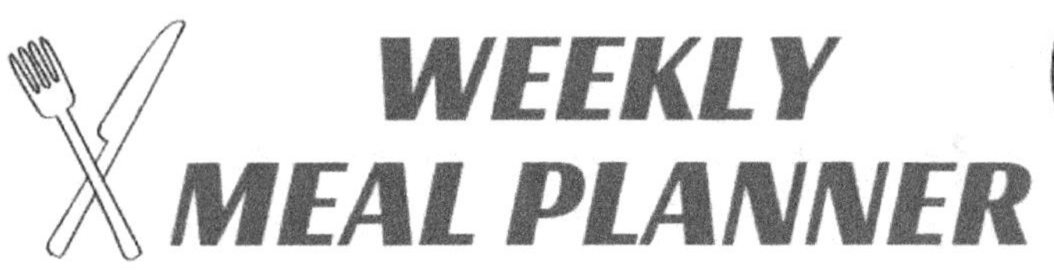

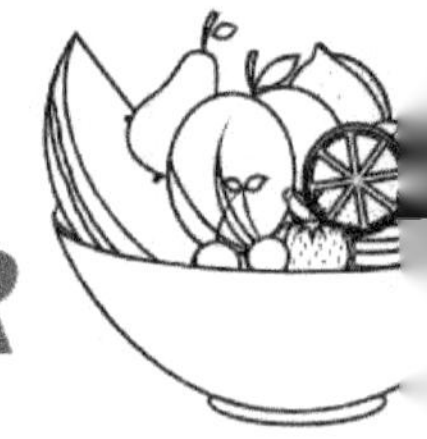

	BREAKFAST	LUNCH	SNACKS	DINNER
MONDAY				
TUESDAY				
WEDNESDAY				
THURSDSAY				
FRIDAY				
SATURDAY				
SUNDAY				

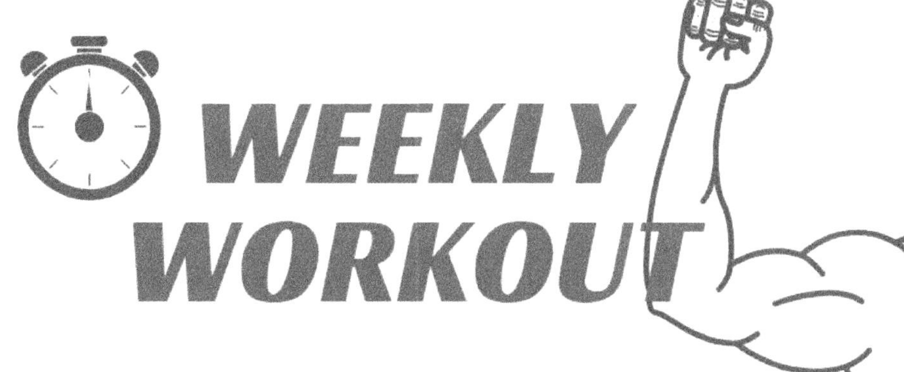

	ACTIVITY	TIME	SETS	REPS
DAY 1				
DAY 2				
DAY 3				
DAY 4				
DAY 5				

GETTING STRONGER EVERY DAY

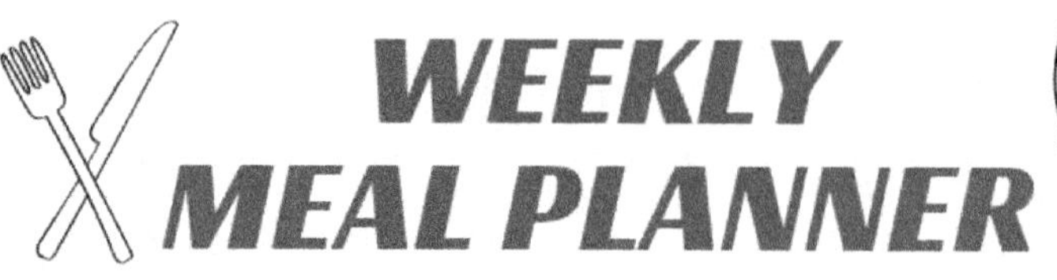

WEEKLY MEAL PLANNER

	BREAKFAST	LUNCH	SNACKS	DINNER
MONDAY				
TUESDAY				
WEDNESDAY				
THURSDSAY				
FRIDAY				
SATURDAY				
SUNDAY				

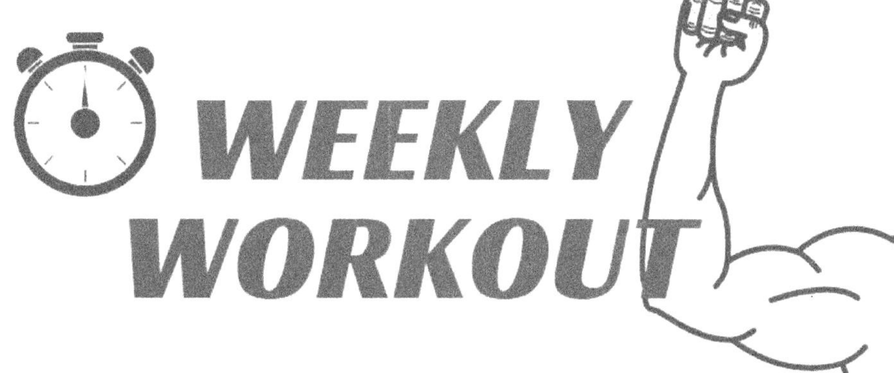

	ACTIVITY	TIME	SETS	REPS
DAY 1				
DAY 2				
DAY 3				
DAY 4				
DAY 5				

GETTING STRONGER EVERY DAY

WEEKLY MEAL PLANNER

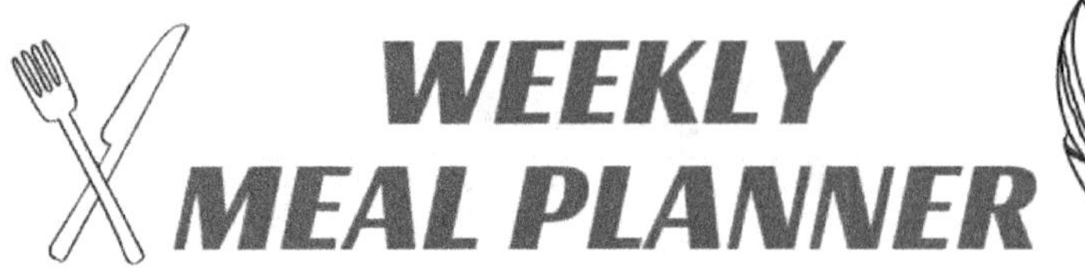

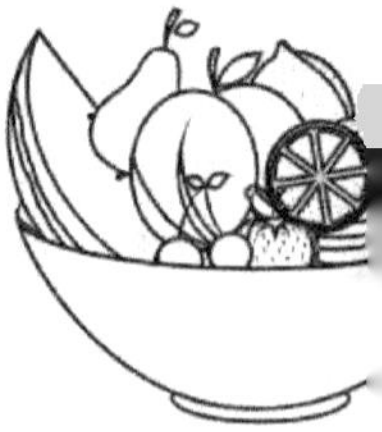

	BREAKFAST	LUNCH	SNACKS	DINNER
MONDAY				
TUESDAY				
WEDNESDAY				
THURSDSAY				
FRIDAY				
SATURDAY				
SUNDAY				

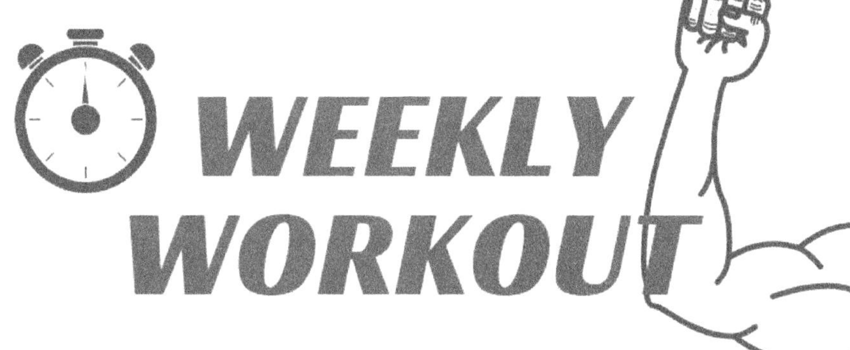

	ACTIVITY	TIME	SETS	REPS
DAY 1				
DAY 2				
DAY 3				
DAY 4				
DAY 5				

GETTING STRONGER EVERY DAY

WEEKLY MEAL PLANNER

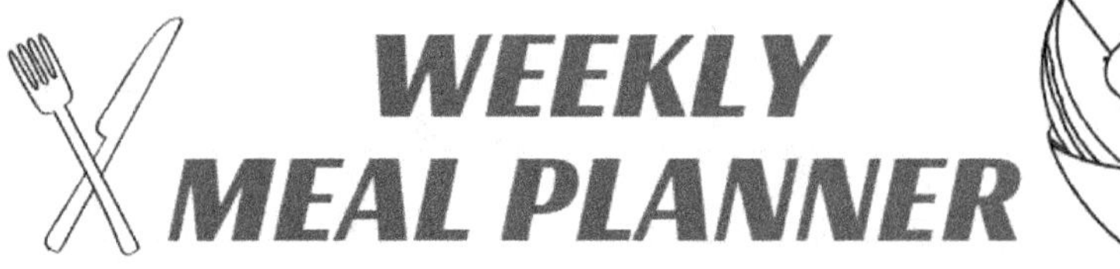

	BREAKFAST	LUNCH	SNACKS	DINNER
MONDAY				
TUESDAY				
WEDNESDAY				
THURSDSAY				
FRIDAY				
SATURDAY				
SUNDAY				

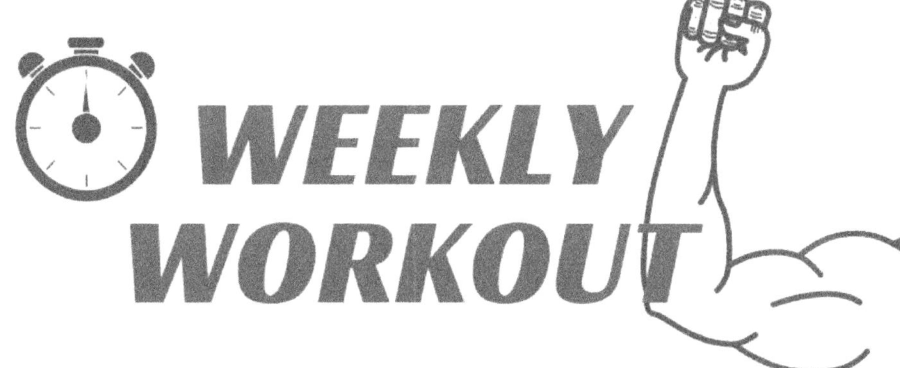

	ACTIVITY	TIME	SETS	REPS
DAY 1				
DAY 2				
DAY 3				
DAY 4				
DAY 5				

GETTING STRONGER EVERY DAY

WEEKLY MEAL PLANNER

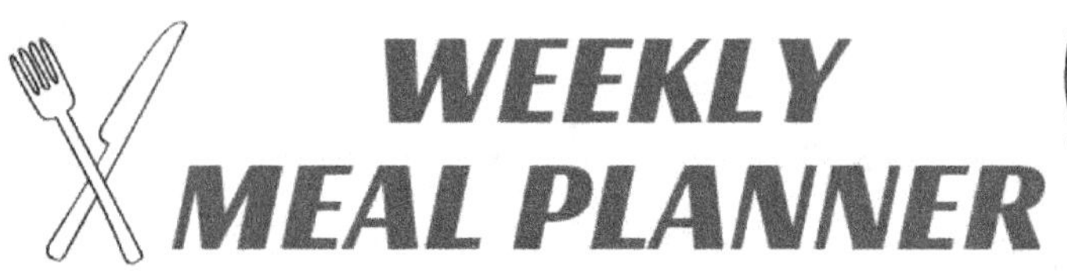
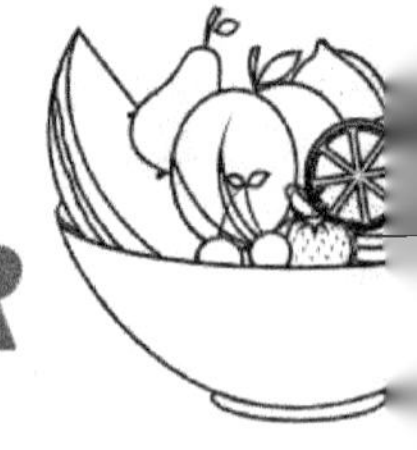

	BREAKFAST	LUNCH	SNACKS	DINNER
MONDAY				
TUESDAY				
WEDNESDAY				
THURSDSAY				
FRIDAY				
SATURDAY				
SUNDAY				

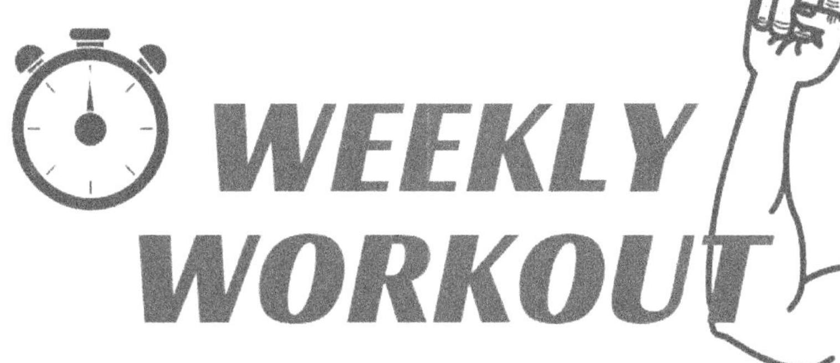

	ACTIVITY	TIME	SETS	REPS
DAY 1				
DAY 2				
DAY 3				
DAY 4				
DAY 5				

GETTING STRONGER EVERY DAY

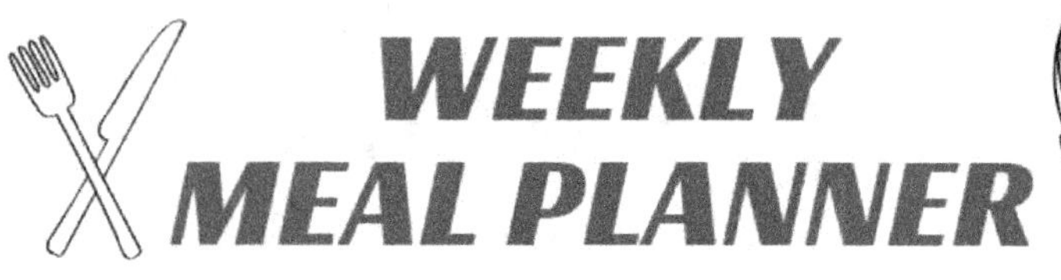

WEEKLY
MEAL PLANNER

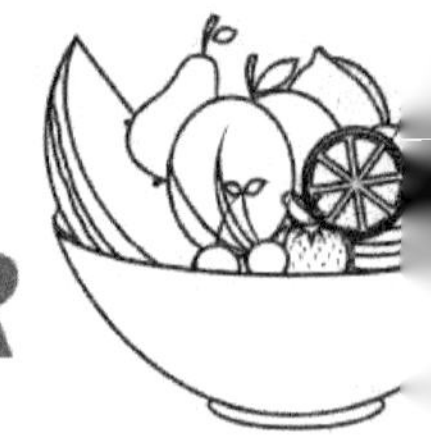

	BREAKFAST	LUNCH	SNACKS	DINNER
MONDAY				
TUESDAY				
WEDNESDAY				
THURSDSAY				
FRIDAY				
SATURDAY				
SUNDAY				

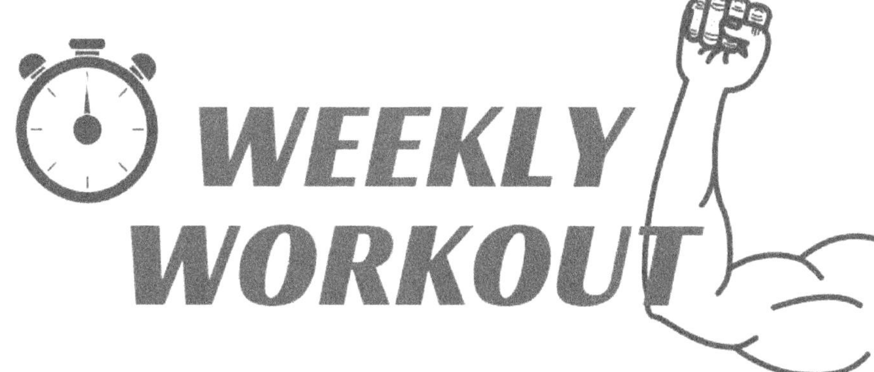

	ACTIVITY	TIME	SETS	REPS
DAY 1				
DAY 2				
DAY 3				
DAY 4				
DAY 5				

GETTING STRONGER EVERY DAY

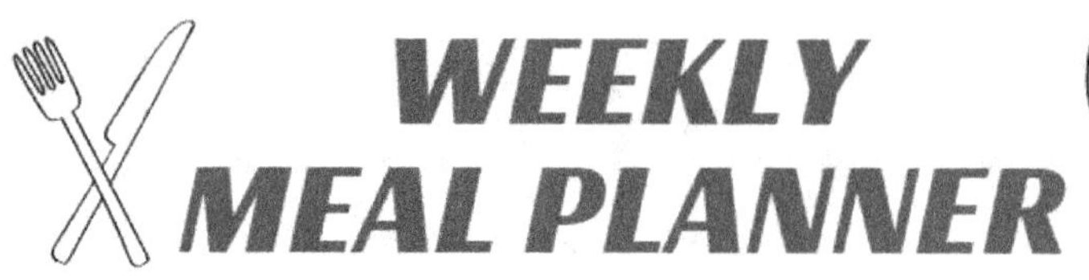

WEEKLY MEAL PLANNER

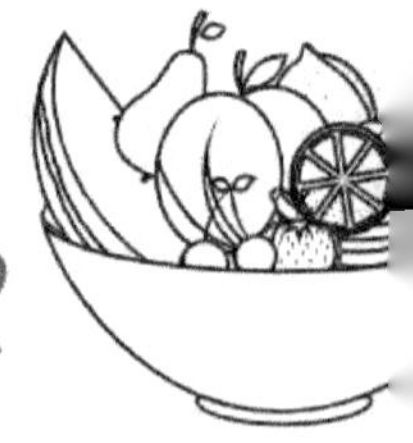

	BREAKFAST	LUNCH	SNACKS	DINNER
MONDAY				
TUESDAY				
WEDNESDAY				
THURSDSAY				
FRIDAY				
SATURDAY				
SUNDAY				

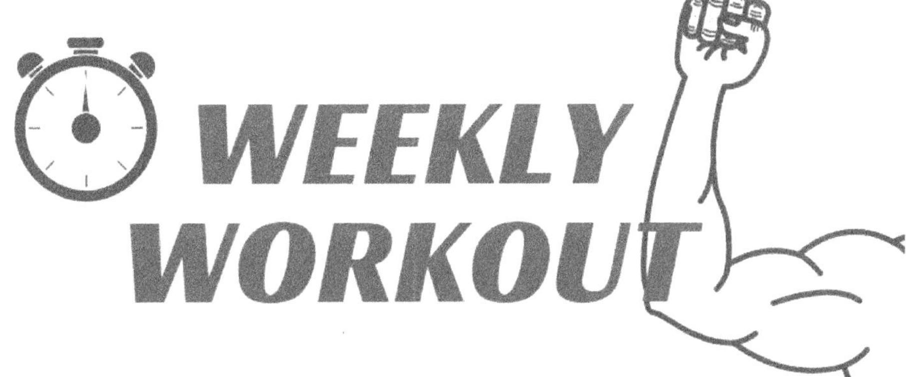

	ACTIVITY	TIME	SETS	REPS
DAY 1				
DAY 2				
DAY 3				
DAY 4				
DAY 5				

GETTING STRONGER EVERY DAY

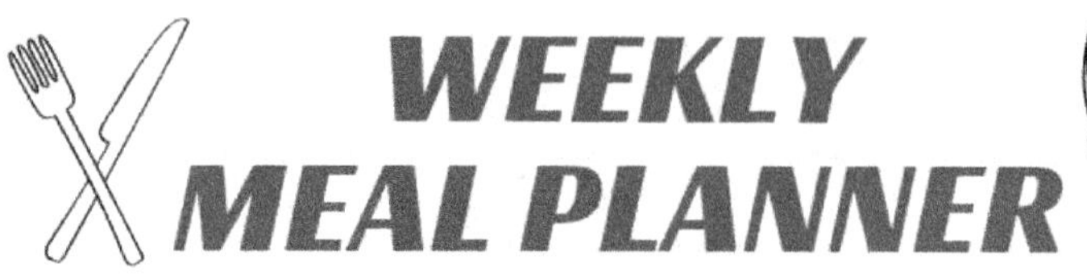

WEEKLY MEAL PLANNER

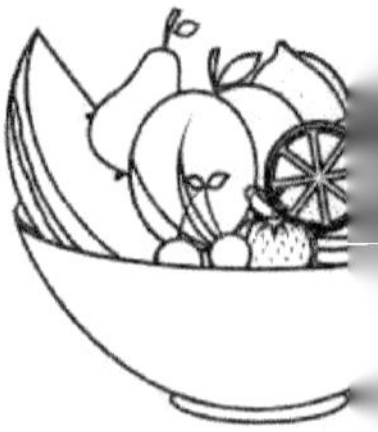

	BREAKFAST	LUNCH	SNACKS	DINNER
MONDAY				
TUESDAY				
WEDNESDAY				
THURSDSAY				
FRIDAY				
SATURDAY				
SUNDAY				

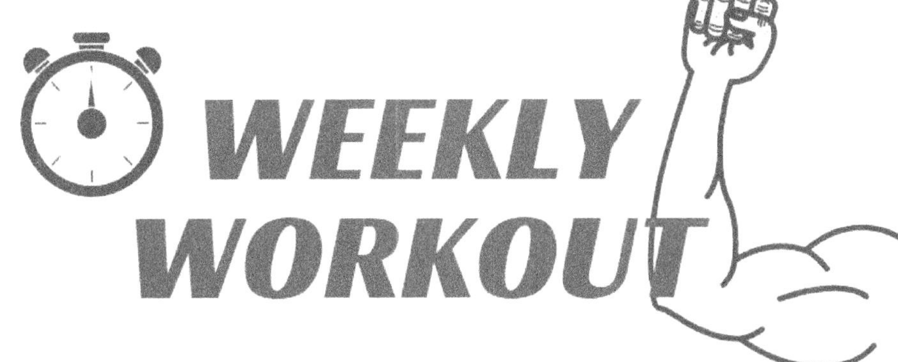

	ACTIVITY	TIME	SETS	REPS
DAY 1				
DAY 2				
DAY 3				
DAY 4				
DAY 5				

GETTING STRONGER EVERY DAY

WEEKLY MEAL PLANNER

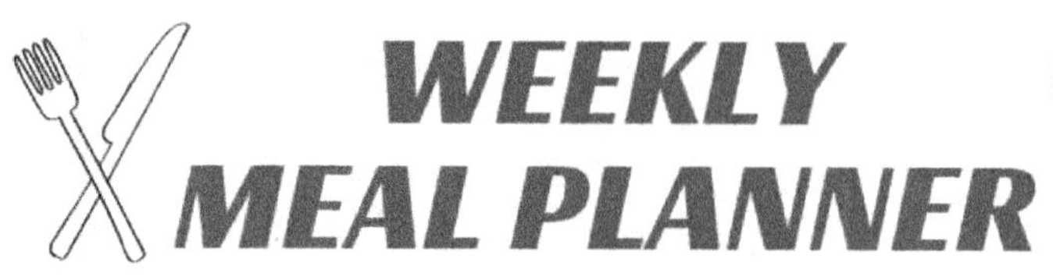

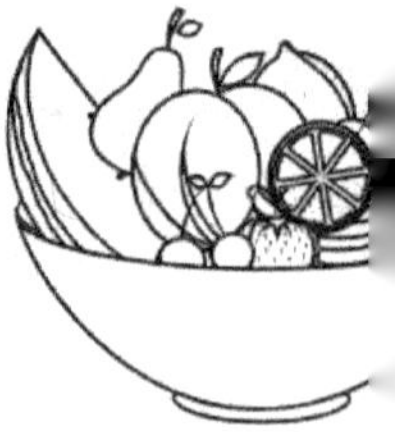

	BREAKFAST	LUNCH	SNACKS	DINNER
MONDAY				
TUESDAY				
WEDNESDAY				
THURSDSAY				
FRIDAY				
SATURDAY				
SUNDAY				

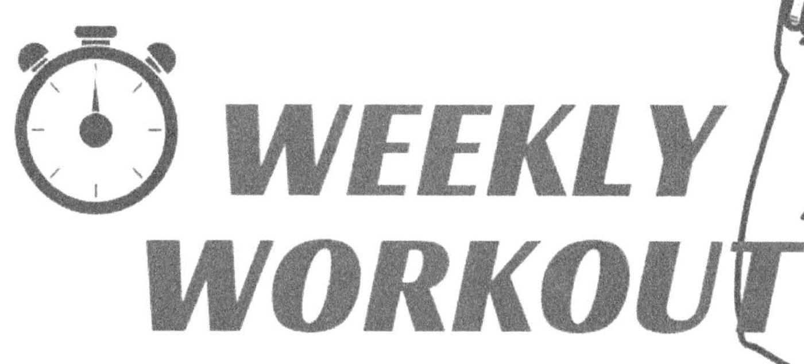

WEEKLY WORKOUT

	ACTIVITY	TIME	SETS	REPS
DAY 1				
DAY 2				
DAY 3				
DAY 4				
DAY 5				

GETTING STRONGER EVERY DAY

WEEKLY MEAL PLANNER

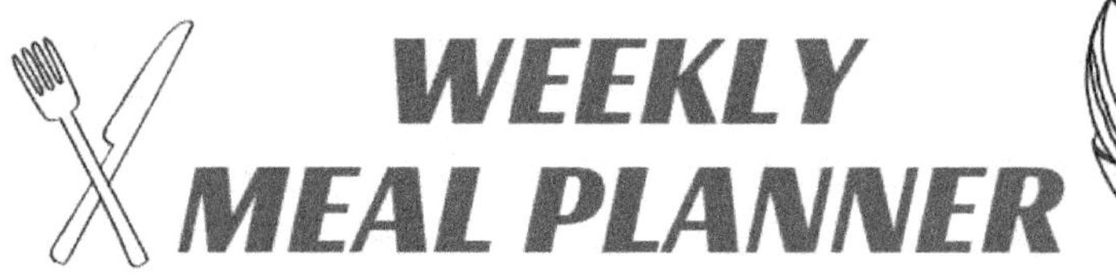

	BREAKFAST	LUNCH	SNACKS	DINNER
MONDAY				
TUESDAY				
WEDNESDAY				
THURSDSAY				
FRIDAY				
SATURDAY				
SUNDAY				

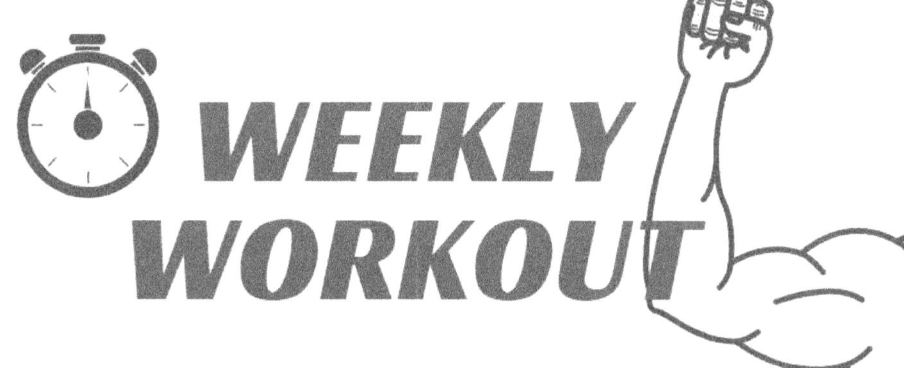

	ACTIVITY	TIME	SETS	REPS
DAY 1				
DAY 2				
DAY 3				
DAY 4				
DAY 5				

GETTING STRONGER EVERY DAY

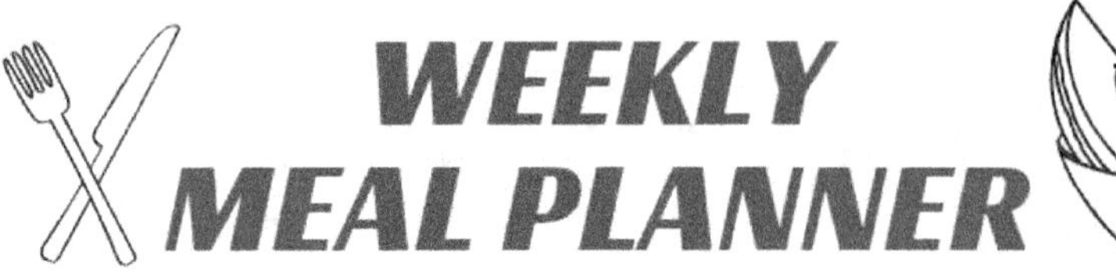

WEEKLY MEAL PLANNER

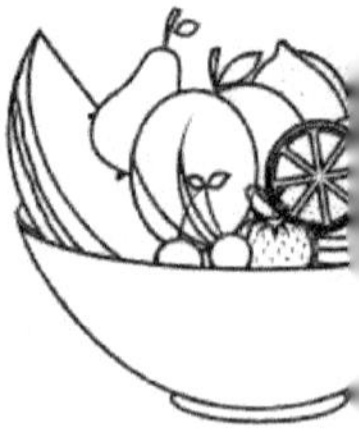

	BREAKFAST	LUNCH	SNACKS	DINNER
MONDAY				
TUESDAY				
WEDNESDAY				
THURSDSAY				
FRIDAY				
SATURDAY				
SUNDAY				

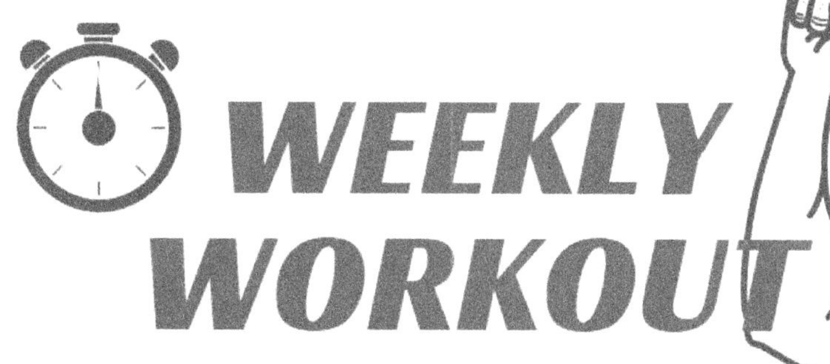

WEEKLY WORKOUT

	ACTIVITY	TIME	SETS	REPS
DAY 1				
DAY 2				
DAY 3				
DAY 4				
DAY 5				

GETTING STRONGER EVERY DAY

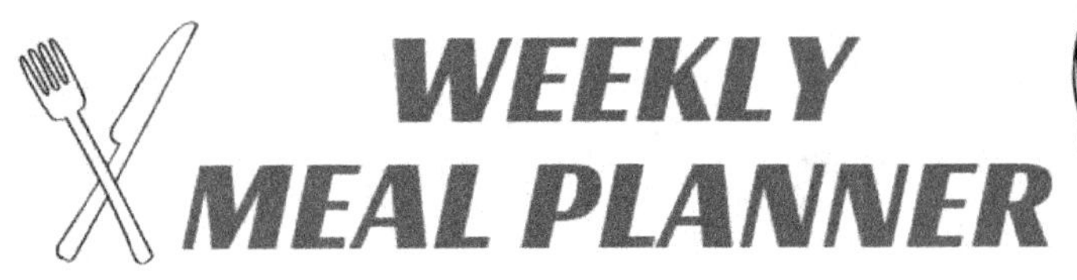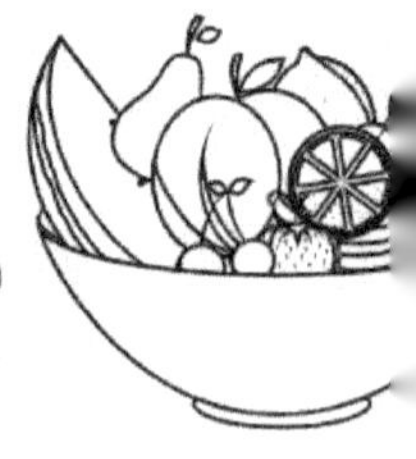

WEEKLY MEAL PLANNER

	BREAKFAST	LUNCH	SNACKS	DINNER
MONDAY				
TUESDAY				
WEDNESDAY				
THURSDSAY				
FRIDAY				
SATURDAY				
SUNDAY				

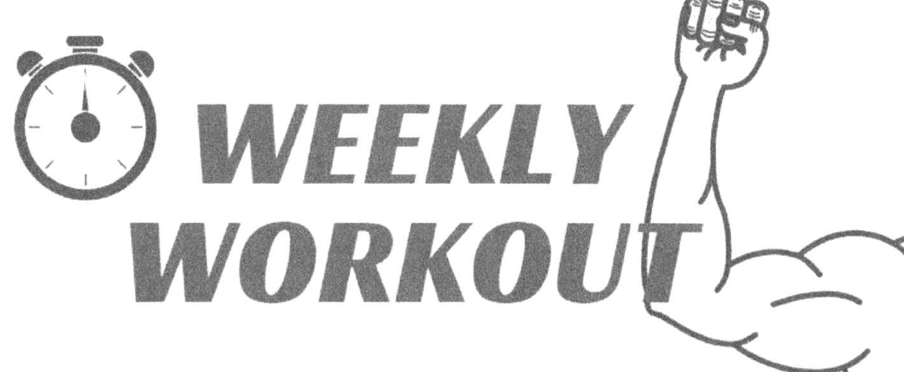

	ACTIVITY	TIME	SETS	REPS
DAY 1				
DAY 2				
DAY 3				
DAY 4				
DAY 5				

GETTING STRONGER EVERY DAY

WEEKLY MEAL PLANNER

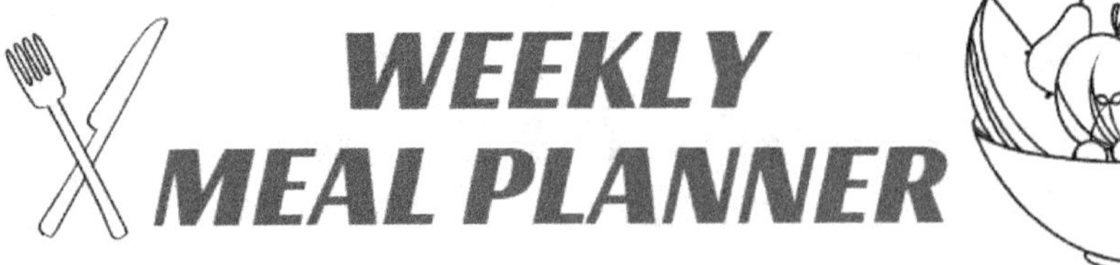

	BREAKFAST	LUNCH	SNACKS	DINNER
MONDAY				
TUESDAY				
WEDNESDAY				
THURSDSAY				
FRIDAY				
SATURDAY				
SUNDAY				

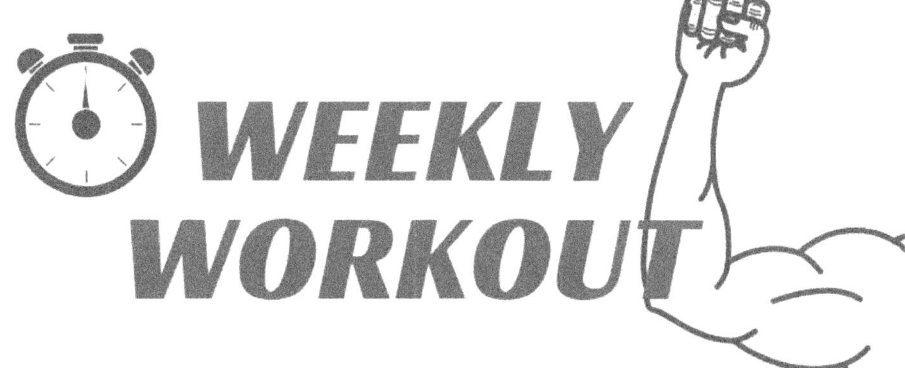

WEEKLY WORKOUT

	ACTIVITY	TIME	SETS	REPS
DAY 1				
DAY 2				
DAY 3				
DAY 4				
DAY 5				

GETTING STRONGER EVERY DAY

WEEKLY MEAL PLANNER

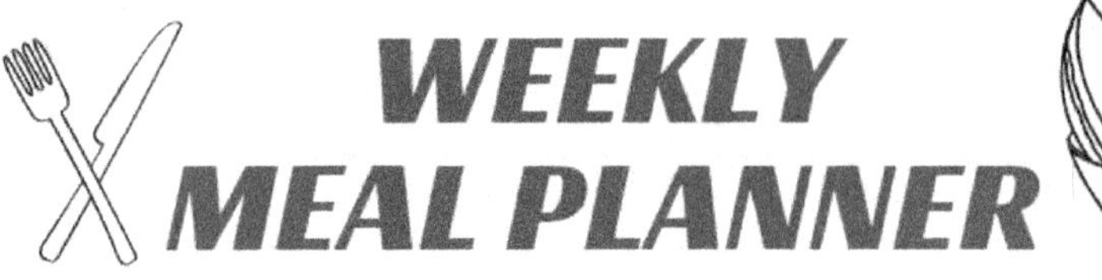

	BREAKFAST	LUNCH	SNACKS	DINNER
MONDAY				
TUESDAY				
WEDNESDAY				
THURSDSAY				
FRIDAY				
SATURDAY				
SUNDAY				

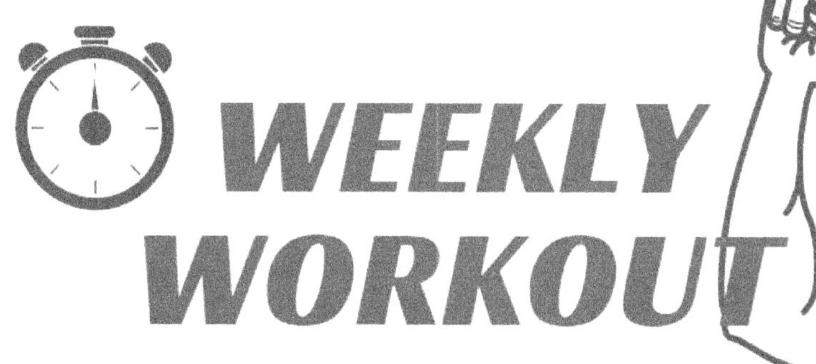

WEEKLY WORKOUT

	ACTIVITY	TIME	SETS	REPS
DAY 1				
DAY 2				
DAY 3				
DAY 4				
DAY 5				

GETTING STRONGER EVERY DAY

WEEKLY MEAL PLANNER

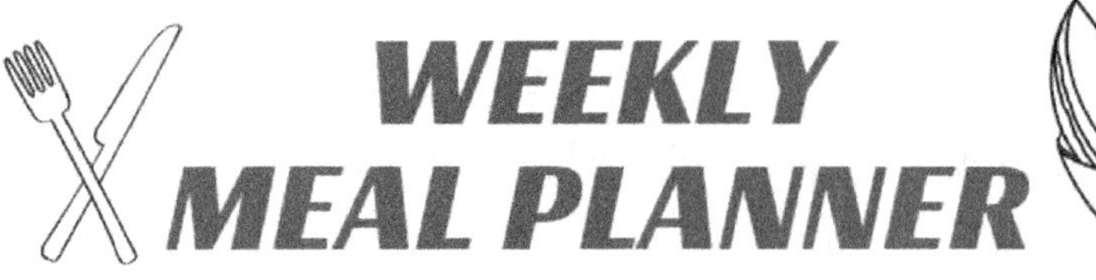

	BREAKFAST	LUNCH	SNACKS	DINNER
MONDAY				
TUESDAY				
WEDNESDAY				
THURSDSAY				
FRIDAY				
SATURDAY				
SUNDAY				

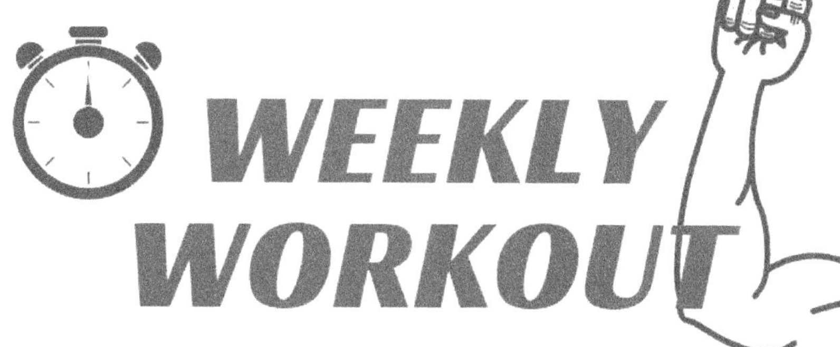

WEEKLY WORKOUT

	ACTIVITY	TIME	SETS	REPS
DAY 1				
DAY 2				
DAY 3				
DAY 4				
DAY 5				

GETTING STRONGER EVERY DAY

www.ingramcontent.com/pod-product-compliance
Lightning Source LLC
Chambersburg PA
CBHW070741250726
48662CB00004B/1609